AFTER A STROKE

AFTER A STROKE

500

TIPS FOR LIVING WELL

Second Edition

By Cleo Hutton

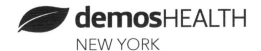

demosHEALTH

NEW YORK

Visit our website at www.demoshealth.com

ISBN: 978-1-936303-96-0
e-book ISBN: 978-1-61705-281-1

Acquisitions Editor: Beth Barry
Compositor: diacriTech

Library of Congress Cataloging-in-Publication Data

Names: Hutton, Cleo, 1949- author.
Title: After a stroke : 500 tips for living well / by Cleo Hutton.
Description: Second edition. | New York, NY : Demos Medical Publishing,
   [2017] | Includes bibliographical references and index.
Identifiers: LCCN 2016024473| ISBN 9781936303960 | ISBN 9781617052811 (ebook)
Subjects: LCSH: Cerebrovascular disease—Popular works.
Classification: LCC RC388.5 .H879 2017 | DDC 616.8/1—dc23 LC record
   available at https://lccn.loc.gov/2016024473

Special discounts on bulk quantities of Demos Health books are available to corporations, professional associations, pharmaceutical companies, health care organizations, and other qualifying groups. For details, please contact:

Special Sales Department
Demos Medical Publishing
11 West 42nd Street, 15th Floor,
New York, NY 10036
Phone: 800-532-8663 or 212-683-0072;
Fax: 212-941-7842
E-mail: specialsales@demosmedpub.com

Printed in the United States of America by McNaughton & Gunn.
16 17 18 19 20 / 5 4 3 2 1

This book is dedicated to my four grandchildren.

You were not yet born when I had the strokes.

Today, I couldn't imagine my life without you.

Contents

Preface

A stroke struck you or someone you love. You have gone through the critical stage of this devastating condition and perhaps even graduated from a hospital rehabilitation program. Now you begin another phase of rehabilitation, as your battle for recovery is showing undeniable progress. You're going home. The purpose of this book is to give you helpful tips and information about stroke that will serve as necessary artillery to empower you to overcome obstacles in the way of successful healing and move forward with your life.

This book offers more than 500 tips for living well after stroke. The tips and information will help you and your family during stroke recovery. Adapt them to your recovery needs, always challenging yourself with new tasks to accomplish. Use what applies to you and your family.

Every tip is numbered. However, you may want to skip ahead or go back to a part in the book that relates to your particular recovery needs. Your needs will change over time. What works for one individual may not be suitable for another. The tips are not presented in order of importance, so you can jump from section to section to find the tips you need on any given day.

I have had several strokes but remain focused on education, medical insight, adaptability, and new techniques in recovery. My goal in writing this book is to relate to other stroke survivors what I have learned and share the tools and best practices that have helped me in my recovery.

Since the 2005 publication of the first edition, significant advances have been made in public education, medical treatment, brain research, and rehabilitation techniques for stroke. Research on brain neuroplasticity—how we learn, how quickly the brain adapts—is rapidly progressing and informing treatment and recovery.

Check with your physician or therapist prior to trying some of the tips. Have a caregiver or family member observe you until you feel comfortable doing a task yourself. Safety and medical supervision are always paramount in successful recovery.

You can live fully after a stroke.

To get you started on that path, here is some general information about stroke and what's happening in the field.

Background

What is stroke?

A stroke happens when the blood supply to part of the brain is interrupted or severely reduced, depriving brain tissue of oxygen and nutrients. Brain cells begin to die within minutes of a stroke, also known as a cerebral vascular accident (CVA). A stroke may be caused by a blocked or narrowed artery (ischemic stroke) or the leaking or bursting of a blood vessel (hemorrhagic stroke). Some people may experience only a temporary interruption of blood flow to their brain, known as a transient ischemic attack (TIA) or mini-stroke.

Ischemic strokes are the most common kind of strokes. Ischemia is the state of reduced blood flow. There are two sub-classes of ischemic stroke: Thrombotic, which happens when a blood clot (thrombus) forms in one of the arteries that supply blood to the brain. This clot may be caused by fatty deposits (plaque) that build up in artery walls causing what is commonly known as "hardening of the arteries" (atherosclerosis). The second sub-class is embolic, which occurs when a blood clot forms in a different part of your body and is carried through your bloodstream eventually plugging narrow brain arteries. An embolism or embolus is the medical term for this second type of blood clot causing an ischemic stroke.

There are two sub-classes of hemorrhagic stroke, as well. During an intracerebral (inside the brain) hemorrhage, a blood vessel in the brain bursts, spilling into the surrounding brain tissue, which can damage cells throughout the brain. The second sub-class is sub-arachnoid hemorrhage, in which an artery near the surface of the brain bursts and spills into the space between the surface of the brain and the skull. This bleeding causes a sudden, severe headache.

A hemorrhagic stroke can be caused by any condition that affects the blood vessels, including uncontrolled high blood pressure (hypertension), overtreatment with anticoagulants (blood thinners), trauma to the brain, and weak spots or pouches in the blood vessel walls (aneurysms). Another cause is the rupture of an abnormal web of thin-walled blood vessels (arteriovenous malformation or AVM) present at birth. After, or during, a hemorrhagic stroke the blood vessels in the brain may intermittently widen and narrow (vaso-spasm), causing further brain cell damage by limiting blood flow. Hemorrhagic strokes are often treated with "clipping" or "coiling" procedures, which reduce blood flow to aneurysms or AVM's.

When one of these types of stroke occur, hospitalization follows. Then begins a rehabilitation process. Therapy is the initial step on the rehabilitation journey.

What's new in hospital treatments?

Tissue plasminogen activator (tPA), a clot-dissolving drug, has proven to be a groundbreaker in the treatment of ischemic type strokes. However, tPA cannot be administered if the patient has had a hemorrhagic stroke. Therefore, it is imperative to diagnose what type of stroke the patient is having before treatment is considered. First, a neurologist observes symptoms and immediately uses mag-netic resonance imaging (MRI), which uses a large magnet and radio waves to produce an image of the brain. A neurologist can use this image to determine what type of stroke has occurred. If the stroke is determined to be ischemic, tPA must be administered within 3 to 4 hours of the onset of stroke symptoms. This means many isch-emic stroke patients do not have the chance to use this treatment; it is estimated that only 4% of these patients receive tPA within this short window of time.

Other medical conditions and/or advanced age could also preclude the use of tPA. This is why stroke prevention and stroke awareness are essential. Because most stroke symptoms are painless—except for hemorrhagic stroke, which can be extremely painful—we tend to downplay the significance of the event. We need to become more aware of how our brain speaks to us. Time, a most precious com-modity when it comes to being treated with tPA, equals the quality of our brain health. The less time it takes in seeking emergency treat-ment for stroke, the less the brain will be affected.

With the advancement of stroke centers, comprehensive stroke centers, technology, and medicine, new treatments are moving for-ward. Among these are new clot-removing devices such as MERCI

Retriever and Penumbra System® MAX™ aspiration system and ACE™ 64 clot extractor. These surgical procedures also must be performed within a relatively short time in order to restore blood flow to the stroke-affected areas in the brain. This technique is currently being used in the United States and Europe.

What's new in stroke rehabilitation?

New rehabilitation techniques now employ technology in therapy by using advanced equipment for arm and leg mobility. Bioness and Saebo are two companies expanding the use of movement of stroke-affected extremities through robotic and wireless technology.

Some therapists in hospitals and rehabilitation centers may use constraint induced therapy (CI or CIMT). This type of therapy restrains the unaffected extremity in order to force neural transmitters to travel and grow around the affected brain areas. In order to use CI therapy, stroke survivors need to be able to extend their wrists and move their arm and fingers. As in any form of therapy, even exercises performed at home, these motions must be repeated until the brain learns to use alternative routes.

Continuation of therapy, at home without therapists to guide you, is vital for neuroplasticity. Hopefully, you were discharged from rehabilitation with an individualized treatment plan. This plan should state what medications you are taking, the dosage, and when to take them, as well as exercises for you to do at home and how often you should do them. It is important to follow your customized treatment plan.

How is the brain affected by stroke?

The brain is complex. Neurotransmitters within the brain are like electrical circuits that travel from one point to another carrying genetic codes, patterns that form our personality, behaviors and emotions, and tell our brain to remember, reason, problem solve, and even instruct our heart to beat and lungs to breathe, among thousands of other duties. When stroke happens, the neurons can no longer get to their destinations. Sometimes the neurons get upset and begin to erratically go off in wrong directions, or misfire, causing seizures. Our brain is as adaptable and as creative as people are when tragedy strikes. In the brain, this is called "plasticity."

Stroke affects every individual differently. This difference is dependent upon the type of stroke (ischemic or hemorrhagic) and the area of the brain affected by the stroke. Just as is true in real estate, "location, location, location" can make all the difference.

Will other medical conditions affect my stroke recovery progress?

Other medical conditions can complicate the recovery process, especially those medical risk factors that may have caused the stroke. These risk factors include heart disease or heart defects, atrial fibrillation (abnormal heart rhythm), high blood pressure (hypertension), high cholesterol, diabetes, smoking, and obstructive sleep apnea (a sleep disorder that causes the oxygen level to sporadically drop during the night, which can result in the forming of a blood clot). Sometimes surgery or a head injury can complicate the recovery process.

There are risk factors we can control, such as weight, physical activity, and the use of alcohol or overuse of medication or drugs. Each of these controllable risk factors will be addressed as we explore various ways to recover from stroke.

As a stroke survivor, you may be aware of the risk factors that cannot be changed, like a family history of stroke, age (55 or older), and race (African Americans have a higher risk of stroke than Caucasians). Sex is a less reliable indicator. A few years ago, males had a higher incidence of stroke. Today, women are leading in stroke occurrences.

Regardless of your background or risk factors, you are now a stroke survivor. The tips in this book are for you.

Acknowledgments

Thank you Beth Kaufman Barry, Publisher, Norman Graubart, Assistant Editor, and the staff at Demos Health for their longstanding dedication to healthy living; especially stroke awareness and recovery.

Thank you also to Jennifer Derrick, writing instructor at the Department of Writing Studies, University of Minnesota Duluth, for assistance with editing and proofreading; to Sheila R. Davidson, MS, CCC/SLP, programs manager for Rehabilitation Services, Essentia Health, Duluth, Minnesota, for steering me in the right direction toward updated therapeutic techniques for stroke survivors; to Christine A. Raso, BA, LSW, STAR/C, case manager at Essentia Health/Polinsky Medical Rehabilitation Center, Duluth, Minnesota, for updated information regarding local and regional stroke support groups; to Henry Hoffman, co-founder of Saebo, for the use of images of Saebo Glove and Saebo Flex/Saebo Reach technology system; to Jeri Francis, senior graphic designer at North Coast Medical, Inc., for the use of images from their Functional Solutions catalog, Volume 7.3; and to Yuri Trejo, principal product manager at Bioness for the use of images of the Ness H200 Wireless and L300 Foot Drop Systems.

Home Recovery

Plateau means we've hit a bump in the road to recovery. It does not mean we have come to the end of the road. On the contrary, our journey has just begun.

The brain is an approximate three-pound part of our central nervous system. It reacts after a head-on collision with stroke. The brain uses a brilliant defense mechanism and goes into a rapid course of plasticity. Temporarily, the brain tries to reorganize itself, like shaking ourselves off after a bad dust storm. The brain tries to recover quickly from the cerebral vascular accident. This is why, in some cases, there may be strides toward recovery in a relatively short time while in therapy.

Unfortunately, the brain has sustained major mechanical damage and begins to run at a slower pace than before. The brain becomes a little less supple or elastic yet has a lot of plasticity remaining to work with and use. The engine is still running, but we don't understand why it isn't humming along like it used to—we have reached a plateau.

Another example of the word "plateau" is when a person desires to lose weight. He or she may join a gym and lose the first five or ten pounds quickly because of the increased activity and focus on healthy eating. The next five pounds will be lost at a slower pace as the body adjusts to the new routine. Eventually, it may become more difficult to lose the extra pounds because the person has plateaued. In order to continue on a weight loss regime, he or she must either exercise at a higher intensity or work out for a longer period of time.

It is possible to get past plateaus, just as it is possible to tune up a car, become a better athlete, or improve countless other skills. The approach in breaking these barriers lies in taking on something new; taking learning to the next level by trying something different. This is the objective behind *After a Stroke: 500 Tips for Living Well*.

1 **Stroke does not define who you are**. If you live entirely absorbed with continuous rehabilitation, you may forget to live. When you finally reach the place where stroke deficits are no longer the first thought you wake up to and your last thought before you sleep at night, you are on your way to living well.

2 **Believe in yourself**. The word "survivor" means you have lived through serious circumstances and survived. In the hospital, rehabilitation unit, or at a stroke support group you may be referred to as a "stroke survivor" and your spouse or family member as your "caregiver." Politically correct language may be appropriate for this setting, but you are home now. You have a name and identity.

3 **If you are continuing outpatient rehabilitation, don't wait until your next session to practice what you've learned**. Brain neurons require constant stimulation in order to make or reroute new connections. It will be more difficult to progress if you depend entirely on formal therapy sessions for your total rehabilitation. You are in charge of teaching those brain neurons to adapt.

4 **Keep trying**. Eventually, you will get to your realistic goals.

Terminology (Tips 5–12)

Relearning language and word definitions can be very challenging after a stroke. How we refer to ourselves and how others vocalize their views can be paramount to our success in stroke recovery. We are not "victims."

5 **Discourage vocabulary such as "good side" or "bad side."** Refer to your right or left side as the "affected side" of your body and the other side as the "unaffected side." The same procedure will be followed throughout this book.

6 **Your family is more than "caregivers."** That is only part of their role. Your family has experienced stroke in a different way than you. Support of all family members is crucial, as stroke is a learning experience for everyone.

7 **"Therapy" is performed in a hospital environment.** You may no longer be in therapy but you are trying to live life to the best of your capabilities and learning new ways of adapting within your home environment.

8 **Independence—stroke survivors need to try to do things for themselves.** We must find our own way of accomplishing daily activities. Love is positive. On the other hand, pampering us with an overabundant amount of attention and doing everything for us will stifle our recovery.

9 **Communication—use concise language and short sentences when speaking to a stroke survivor with aphasia.** Aphasia is a condition that may occur after a stroke, taking away the ability to communicate. Various forms of aphasia affect the ability to speak, write, or understand verbal or written language. Many stroke survivors cannot remember or integrate long dialogues. Concrete, simple concepts may be easier to understand when recovering from stroke. Say what you mean, as we relearn the spoken word.

10 **Comprehension—speak to us in a normal tone and with normal voice inflection**. We can hear the words but may have difficulty in comprehending the meaning.

11 **Speech—recognize and address communication difficulties**. Some stroke survivors have relearned to speak but may become verbose. This condition is common with a right-sided brain injury. The language and speech centers may have been affected. Speech therapy is vitally important for relearning speech. Also, exposure to language is important. A lack of language skills can lead to isolation, depression, overstimulation, loss of independence, and misunderstandings.

12 **Language—we may use inappropriate language**. Some stroke survivors may use inappropriate language even if they have never used this language before the stroke. This may happen because most expletive-deleted words are monosyllabic and easier to speak, especially when frustrated. Our caregivers need to know that we may say an inappropriate word but mean something entirely different. They need to be patient with us as we attempt to find our language abilities.

Reading and Comprehension (Tips 13–21)

If stroke has affected your vision and comprehension skills, here are some helpful tools to aid in relearning the written word.

"Stop, right there! How can we read when we can't see the entire page? (visual field deficit) or the many other visual problems that can come with stroke, like alexia (complete impairment of the ability to read)?" Good question. You are addressing visual perceptual processing. We can't process what we don't see. Therefore, for stroke survivors with alexia, I am hopeful that a family member is reading this book to them. For stroke survivors who have visual field difficulties there is a two-word answer that is interwoven throughout this book—"spatial retraining." This process stimulates thinking (cognitive) development. Repetition of games, puzzles, object recognition, conversations with loved ones, social skills, relearning to see objects on your affected side, mirrors, hobbies such as painting or drawing, using a computer, exercising, and more add up to stimulating the visual field.

If you are unable to read due to alexia, try the next three tips. If you have difficulty with visual field, try tips 16 to 21.

13 **Use a small tape recorder and, with the permission of people who are speaking, tape vital conversations**. In the hospital, this technique assisted my family in listening to physician's conversations and helped me remember information. In the classroom, with each professor's permission, this system worked well to tape lectures so I could replay the tape several times to improve comprehension and memory skills. Sometimes, old technology remains useful (though a smartphone will work, too).

14 **Use audio books or books on compact discs (CDs)**. Audio books can be ordered online or purchased through bookstores. Comprehension skills can be developed through listening.

15 **Consider the National Library Service (NLS) for digital audiobooks, large-print books, and online formats that will help you in auditory learning**. This service is free to those who qualify. This is a service of the Library of Congress. The NLS contains fiction, nonfiction, bestsellers, classics, biographies, romance novels, music, instructional material, and magazines and material is available in Spanish as well. It is listed in the "Resources" section of this book.

16 **Keep reading**. Reading and comprehension may be difficult after a stroke because other areas of our brain must take over for the stroke-affected areas. There are several ways to re-route those neurons. Since reading and comprehension are of primary importance to everyday living, let's begin with some uncomplicated tasks and work toward more challenging skills.

17 **Use a large print book while listening to an audio version, and follow each word with your finger or a piece of paper.** Looking at the printed words while hearing them read will reinforce language and remind you to move your head and eyes to the end of the page to catch all the text.

18 **Use a magnifying glass or enlargement reader.** An enlargement reader can be purchased through many special equipment catalogues. Another place to obtain a magnification reader is through North Coast Medical at 800-821-9319 or online at www.ncmedical.com. The magnification reader in the accompanying image is featured in the North Coast Medical Functional Solutions catalog.

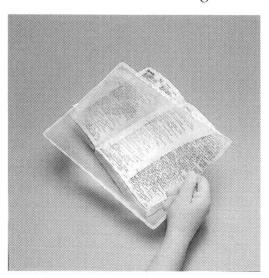

19 **Use technology to assist in reading and comprehension skills.** Use computer programs that allow you to increase the font size for readability. Technology also allows you to connect with other stroke survivors on social network sites available through your smartphone or computer. Even old technology can be used to your advantage. Use the closed caption feature on your television for word recognition while simultaneously hearing the audio.

20   **Read one sentence at a time**. Then, stop reading. Try to visualize the meaning of the sentence. At first, this procedure is very time-consuming and tiring. Rest. Go back to the project when you are ready. You are building new neuron pathways in your brain.

21   **If you own a large print book, draw a red line down the margin of the side of the page corresponding to your affected visual field**. This will remind you to go back to the red line to catch the entire sentence.

Emotional Lability/Pseudobulbar Affect (Tips 22–24)

After a stroke, emotional responses may be affected. Emotional lability and pseudobulbar affect (PBA) are synonymous in describing sudden uncontrollable laughing or crying for no apparent reason or at inappropriate times.

22   **You have a right to know and learn what area(s) the stroke affected and the functions of those areas.** Knowing will provide insight regarding how to compensate, adapt, and eventually overcome the impact of stroke. Your physician will show you your magnetic resonance image (MRI) and relate this information to you. Request permission to record his or her explanation to compensate for your memory difficulties and add to your recovery-learning process. The more factual information we know about our medical history, the less anxious we will feel. The adage "knowledge is power" is paramount to stroke recovery.

23   **Emotional lability/PBA is caused by the stroke**. Many stroke survivors feel ashamed or isolate themselves from others because of PBA. More and more national attention is being called to this side effect of stroke through television public service announcements and magazine articles. Being afraid or ashamed of something we have no control over is like trying to stop a speeding train with a feather. Your tears and laughter will subside to an appropriate level. Antidepressants are not always the best alternative for all stroke survivors as a sure-fire cure for PBA. Your emotions are hyperactive because the stroke affected them.

24 **PBA can be explained to visitors who may not be aware of difficulties with emotional responses if it becomes necessary to do so.** Isolation is not the answer to dealing with PBA. If inappropriate emotional outbursts crop up when friends are around, your friends won't run away in fear.

Posttraumatic Stress Disorder (Tips 25 and 26)

Posttraumatic stress disorder (PTSD) is a psychological reaction that occurs after a stressful event. Stroke is a sudden stressful event. Recurring memories of the traumatic event cause anxiety and fear. The "What if it happens again?" fear can be overwhelming for stroke survivors. The continuous mental loop of real or imagined memories can cause flashbacks and nightmares. Many stroke survivors recall in detail the day they had the stroke. They know the date and partially what occurred because of what they remember or what others have told them.

Imagine memory as a computer in which we extract a file, edit, and return, instead of a book in a library where we pull it out, read it, and put it back. By recalling this computer file, we continuously reinforce an unpleasant memory; possibly because it was so life changing. Our brain may be trying to make sense of the event. This is where yoga, meditation, guided imagery, and mindfulness training are most helpful. These techniques help us to quiet and clear the mind and focus on the present moment, our breathing, and our body.

25 **PTSD is associated with stroke because stroke is a sudden traumatic change.** Stroke is something we cannot get over quickly. It is a life-changing event that we will always remember. Hopefully, in time, those memories will not be as vivid. We will be able to replace some of the bad memories with good ones.

26 **Visual agnosia may lead to symptomatic PTSD or PBA.** Most people take seeing, recognition, and verbal responses for granted. If shown a picture of a key for a door, for example, most people would know it was a key. This may not be a simple matter after a stroke. A stroke survivor may know what it is and what it does but may be unable to recall the name of the object. It is important to address a condition called "visual agnosia" (a stroke affecting the visual association cortex of the brain causing the inability to recognize familiar objects). A stroke survivor may be trying to access that file in his or her mental computer that has the name "key," but the computer freezes. This difficulty can cause problems in everyday living as well. It is a frightening and frustrating experience to see something—an object or a person—and not be able to recognize what or who it is. We know in our hearts and minds what something is and just can't recall the simple name. Sometimes, stroke survivors may be working so hard at trying to recall the name of an object or person that they cascade into an episode of PTSD or PBA. It is difficult to slow down and take the time necessary for the brain to heal and make new connections when we live in a fast-paced world. Most stroke survivors with visual agnosia will improve with time and patience.

Depression (Tips 27–41)

27 **Consult with your neurologist regarding medications for depression or to help combat emotional lability/PBA.** Antidepressant medication should be given on a case-by-case basis.

28 **Acknowledging depression and using various tools to manage depression is key to our recovery**. Depression can begin directly after stroke, or weeks or even years later. Some individuals had depression, either diagnosed or undiagnosed, before having a stroke. Depression impacts the quality of life, and therefore stunts the progression of stroke recovery. The complexity and suddenness of stroke carries a life-changing effect to our lives. Everything has changed: our senses, our ability or inability to communicate, our thinking, our memory, our ability to move, our relationships, our finances, the list goes on. Depression has a huge impact on stroke recovery.

29 **Watch for the symptoms of depression**. They include feelings of helplessness, hopelessness, overwhelming sadness, loss of interest in once pleasurable experiences or activities, excessive tiredness or the inability to sleep, and suicidal tendencies. It seems that depression and stroke walk hand-in-hand. There are very few stroke survivors who have escaped the grasp of depression.

30 **After a stroke, it is normal to feel angry, frustrated, sad, fearful, and anxious**. If these emotions do not subside, medical intervention is necessary. Because of the many aspects of stroke, a variety of treatments or management tools are available.

31 **Any time depression strikes, one alternative is talk therapy**. This takes place with a psychologist or neuropsychologist, and is highly recommended.

32 **Antidepressant medication can be given to help counteract depression**. Sometimes, various medications will have to be tried over months of treatment until you feel improvement. Other strategies can also help and will be addressed in various chapters.

33 **Ask your physician to check your blood chemistry for vitamin deficiencies, anemia, and folic acid deficiencies**. Depression could stem from low blood chemistry as well.

34 **Request a nutrition plan from your physician, stroke support team member, or a certified nutritionist.** Improving eating habits will go a long way in fighting depression.

35 **Attend a stroke support group.** Most rehabilitation facilities or area hospitals offer monthly group meetings for stroke survivors.

36 **Set and prioritize realistic goals.** Accomplishing tasks will help you feel stronger and more independent.

37 **Practice daily stress management.** Gentle yoga, mindfulness therapeutic techniques, aromatherapy, guided imagery, meditation, journaling, or a short walk outside are extremely helpful in fighting depression.

38 **Community involvement is key to battling depression.** The more you are with others, the less you will be thinking about stroke. Volunteer or join a club or group in your neighborhood.

39 **Exercise.** The more you get out of the house and get involved with a wellness or health and fitness center, the better you will feel about yourself. Even if you use adaptive aids, you can attend a low impact or swimming class in your community.

40 **Educate yourself.** Attend a community college or college class or a college for seniors workshop offered in your community. Check with an educational facility or the Department of Rehabilitation Services in your city for tuition grant requirements. This step fights depression, not only by getting you out of the house, but by keeping your mind active on a subject that interests you.

41 **Eliminate alcohol consumption.** Alcohol is a depressant.

Today, addressing issues such as PBA, PTSD, and depression are integral parts of stroke recovery. Neurophysiologists or psychologists usually consult with stroke survivors and their families before the patient is sent home.

Rest (Tips 42–47)

Stroke recovery will not happen in a day, week, month, or year. It is a slow process that necessitates work as well as rest. You are better today than you were yesterday and you will continue to improve as you work toward your recovery.

42 **Your attitude and effort will impact your recovery process.** Giving up is not an option; rest coupled with exercise is the best alternative.

43 **Alternate exercise or activity with rest periods.** Your energy level will be lessened directly after stroke.

44 **You may tire easily and your body and brain may demand frequent naps.** Listen to your body.

45 **Too much sleep leads to depression.** Gauge rest periods around stimulating activities that challenge your concentration skills and exercise your body.

46 **Work at tolerating longer periods of wakefulness.** However, balance it with at least one nap in the afternoon.

47 **A "power nap" is necessary for most stroke survivors, no matter what age they are.** The brain is like a large rechargeable battery. When it drains of power, you tire and your stroke-affected side begins to weaken more than usual. You may trip on your affected foot or droop to one side when sitting erect. Your body and brain are telling you to rest. A short nap recharges your brain battery enough to keep you up and active.

Anger Versus Rage (Tips 48–52)

Anger can be a wonderful motivator. It is the first cousin, Rage, that we need to shy away from. Rage has no boundaries. Rage has no point except pure frustration. Rage will drain you of your power over stroke. Rage is frightening to yourself and others.

Anger can motivate you to get out of bed to let the cat or dog out, get dressed, or even tie your shoes no matter how much time it takes to do so. Anger may assist you with fighting complacency. As long as anger is not directed at another person or yourself and is used solely for motivation, anger can be a good emotion.

48   **Use anger wisely**. Anger may help you to perform a task when you are well rested.

49   **Make sure safety issues are in place**. This is important before attempting a task, especially when you are angry.

50   **Time is your advocate, not your adversary**. Frequently, we get angry because healing from stroke isn't occurring fast enough or on our schedule. So we wait. The act of sitting or staying in bed waiting for healing to just happen on its own leads to depression, weak muscles, pain or severe discomfort on your stroke-affected side, spasticity (involuntary muscle contractions or tightening), and shoulder subluxation (abnormal position of the shoulder)—more about spasticity and subluxation of shoulder are discussed in the "Spasticity and Shoulder Subluxation" (tips 97–105) section. It is a natural response to care for ourselves after a long hospitalization. But time is our enemy when we realize we are missing out on living.

51   **Anger is a normal response; rage must be controlled**. Everyone gets angry occasionally. Rage can be characterized as an uncontrollable, violent, and intense form of anger that can manifest into screaming, yelling, or a fit of explosive bottled-up frustration.

52 Try to verbally express how you are feeling. If words are difficult; take time out to rest your body and mind until the feeling subsides. Then, start again.

Adaptation (Tips 53–64)

Teamwork is essential after a stroke. Medical personnel worked as a team while you were hospitalized. At home, you and your family are the stroke team. An encouraging cheering section does a world of good toward your improvement.

It is important that your home is also adapted to meet your needs. Safety, accessibility, and independence are three priorities.

53 Accept help only when necessary. We feel helpless after stroke. Our first inclination is to have everyone around us assist us in getting better. Stroke survivors move from the hospital where food is prepared and served to them, assistance is provided day and night, proper safety precautions are taken, and medications are brought to them, to a home environment where they have to do everything themselves; again, another shock to our system as we realize the difficulty of this self-sustaining task.

Our nemesis, depression, may be rearing its ugly head. The statement, "I can't!" is usually followed by "You don't understand!"

A new strategy is needed. Perhaps something like, "I will try (getting dressed, folding towels or matching socks, making the bed, or whatever easy task you think you can accomplish) but I need help with preparing my daily medications."

54 Stroke survivors who have aphasia (loss of ability to understand, speak, read, and/or write) should not be left home alone.

55 Accept assistance when you feel uncomfortable doing something yourself. There is a first time for everything. If a family member or caregiver is there to "spot" you the first time you do a task yourself, you may feel more comfortable and confident about your recovery process.

56 Eliminate throw rugs. They could cause a stroke survivor to trip and fall.

57 Wear comfortable clothes and always wear your shoes and ankle-foot orthotic (AFO) when up and about. Comfort and adaptability are key to your success.

58 Install handrails on both sides of stairways. One is for going up and the other for coming down. One side of your body may be weaker than the other.

59 Rearrange furniture so that you can move freely. You will need assistance with this tip. If you are using an adaptive aid like a walker or cane, you need room to move safely and comfortably from one place to another.

60 A ramp may be necessary for any steps outside your home. There are community organizations that charge a nominal fee (or nothing at all) to install a certified handicap ramp for you. Start by contacting your local senior citizen group or disability services offered within your community for referrals.

61 Doors can be removed to allow for wider entry space. Check your doorways for space for your adaptive aids. This is a temporary solution as you may not have to use adaptive aids forever.

62 Avoid chairs that have wheels on the base. This may seem like common sense but it is mentioned to alert stroke survivors to notice the legs of a chair before attempting to sit down.

63 **Sit on a chair at the kitchen table when you are preparing food**. If you don't have a kitchen table, use the counter and sit on a sturdy chair. You may have to purchase one that is solid, safe, and comfortable.

64 **Move items that you use frequently within your reach**. Again, this seems like common sense but it avoids the frustration of having to find things and then, quite possibly, forgetting what you're looking for in the first place. Short-term memory loss can be a side effect of stroke.

Adaptive Aids (Tips 65–82)

There may come a time that you think you can do more than you are able to perform safely. Falls usually injure the stroke-affected side of the body because you may have little to no reaction time to protect your stroke-affected side. In some cases, you may not realize the extent of an injury because the stroke has interrupted pain receptors. Walkers, canes, and braces are used for support, movement, and safety while you are recovering.

65 **Purchase or rent only the equipment you need for your adaptive lifestyle now**. You may improve in time. You may find an easier way to perform a task.

66 **What do you need to do the task safely?** Your adaptive aids will vary. Balance safety with needs. By trying to do various tasks in different ways you are working the brain. With safety as your guideline, try to bring your thought processes to a proper conclusion. One plus two does not always equal three after a stroke. Perhaps think one, and another one, and another one, slowly reaching the same conclusion but adapting to your learning style.

67 **Thrombi embolism disease (TED) stockings** fit snugly against your legs to prevent swelling. There are adaptive aids available to help you put them on and take them off. (The accompanying image shows a two-handed device because it is important to use your stroke-affected hand as much as possible.) Compression stockings will be part of most stroke survivors' daily uniform, especially during the first year when your activity level is lower than normal. Make sure you wear them especially when you are traveling a long distance in a car or in an airplane as airline cabin pressure can cause severe swelling in your legs.

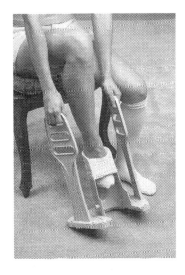

Some items that may be useful to you when getting dressed are as follows:

68 **Elastic waistbands** on slacks, pants, or skirts;

69 **Pullover shirts and sweaters that are a size larger than you normally wear;**

70 **Earrings with metal wires that snap into back fasteners** will be easier to wear than post earrings;

71 **Shoes with Velcro closures or elastic or coiled-elastic shoe-laces** that can be pulled closed but do not need to be tied;

72 **Button hooks** when wearing clothing with small buttons;

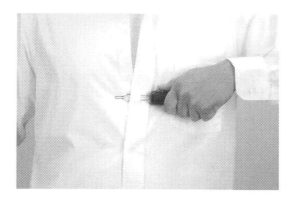

73 **Zippered jackets or other clothing items, with a string** attached through the hole at the end of the zipper for easier reach and closure;

74 **For women: sports bras** that fit over the head or **front closure brassieres;**

75 **A long shoe horn** for putting on your shoes without bending down.

Handy Kitchenware Items

76 **A rocking knife** for easier food cutting using one hand (available through North Coast Medical, Inc., listed in the "Resources" section of this book);

77 **A rolling cart** for easy food preparation and to hold commonly used objects;

78 **A dishwasher safe cutting board with suction cup feet and a vise grip** for safely and easily slicing, dicing, mincing, or chopping food (see more about this device in the "Cooking" section of Chapter 5, tips 217–233; a food processor works well too);

79 A jar and can opener that you can use one handed (there are several styles to choose from in adaptability catalogs);

80 Tongs of various lengths: long-handled salad tongs, ice tongs, or anything that is fastened together and has a large gripping surface and good hand support;

81 Colored foam tubing that builds up cutlery and other handles to make them easier to grasp with your stroke-affected hand.

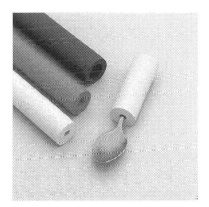

Miscellaneous Adaptive Aid

82 Place your watch on the wrist of your affected side. Use a leather band type with a buckle and place the watch dial on your wrist, flip your wrist over and lay it on a flat surface and buckle it with your unaffected hand. When you want to see the time, you must learn to recognize your affected side.

Medications (Tips 83–96)

83 Take your medication as directed. When to take your medication is just as important as what type of medication it is. Are you to take it with food for better absorption, or on an empty stomach so it doesn't mix with food? Are you to take it before bed because it makes you sleepy, or three times a day spaced morning, noon, and night? Does your medication state "could cause drowsiness"? Less activity is advised after taking the dosage including driving which will be addressed in Chapter 6. These are important signals because the strength, or how your body uses the medication, will be decreased or increased by improper use.

84 **Make sure every physician, pharmacist, and dentist you visit is aware of every medication and over-the-counter (OTC) remedy or medicine you are taking.** Side effects can happen if medical personnel are not aware of everything you take; all the prescribed, as well as OTC, herbal and health store supplements.

85 **Take current medication information with you when visiting physicians, dentists, and pharmacists.** Enter information regarding every medication you are taking, and any supplements, into your computer, or request a family member to do it for you. Type in the name of the medication or product, dosage or strength, times it should be taken, and the reason you are taking it.

86 **Your pharmacist will be another line of defense against side effects,** provided you use the same pharmacy each time you fill or refill prescriptions.

87 **Taking OTC medication without checking with your physician first could cause a lack of potency or side effect when mixed with another medication you are taking.** Even a simple cold remedy, herbal supplement, or high-potency vitamin can cause problems. For instance, if you're prescribed a blood-thinning medication, like Coumadin, and you decide to take aspirin too, this could cause internal bleeding as they are not to be taken together. Another example is taking tonic water for leg cramps. Tonic water is a derivative of quinine and should not be taken if you are taking any type of blood thinners, especially Coumadin, as it could cause internal bleeding.

88 **Food choices may have to be altered with the medication you take**. Again, check with your physician for any written material regarding what to avoid while taking a certain medication.

89 **Take your medications on time and as directed**. Most prescribed medication comes with an insert about side effects. It is important to keep these inserts in a file so you can refer back to them if you are having difficulty. The insert will also explain what you should do if you miss a dose and how to get back on track with the medication. Some medication is to be taken with food. This should be stated on the medication container.

90 **Never stop taking a medication unless your physician has instructed you to do so**. Some medications may take time to build up in your system to work properly. Others may cause negative reactions if stopped abruptly; antidepressants are an example.

91 **Place medications that don't require refrigeration in a drawer with a lock, or in a container that has a lock that only you and other adults can operate**.

92 If you do tip 91 then you may **request that your medication lids be flipped over so that they are easier to open** versus child proof caps. Make it easy on yourself but difficult for children.

93 **Request bold print on medication labels for easier reading**.

94 **If you have difficulty swallowing, request a liquid form of the medication**, or try tucking your chin to your chest when swallowing. Sometimes, pills need to be ground up and taken with easy-to-swallow food.

95 **Take your medications with you on day trips or vacations**. When traveling, carry your medications on your person; in your purse or back pack. Bring an emergency card containing your physician's name, contact number, and all medications you are currently taking. Never pack medications in your luggage. The luggage may be lost, resulting in one or several missed doses. If you are diabetic, you are aware of equipment needed for checking glucose levels and your necessary medication. When traveling, make sure you have water and food available when taking medications.

96 **BlinkHealth.com is an alternative to costly co-pays for necessary medication(s)**. Whether you have insurance or not, this website bypasses insurance co-pays. Before going to the pharmacy, visit www.BlinkHealth.com, enter your prescription as well as dosage and quantity, check to see if the pharmacy you use is part of the BlinkHealth.com network by entering your zip code, prepay for your prescription online, receive a digital copy of your prepaid voucher, take the voucher and your prescription to your local pharmacy. BlinkHealth.com is not an insurance company or a pharmacy. Rather, it is a free and accessible website where you can search for low-cost generic medication without the variable or high cost of co-pay insurance. It may be worthwhile checking this site to see if you can get your prescribed medication at a lower cost.

There are other companies that provide this service as well. Good Rx is another. They quote you generic drug prices directly from pharmaceutical companies and the consumer purchases a coupon to take to the pharmacist. Co-pays are not accepted if you decide to use this alternative.

Spasticity and Shoulder Subluxation (Tips 97–105)

What Is Spasticity?

A stroke may cause muscles on your affected side to involuntarily contract by shortening or flexing when you try to move the affected limb. The limbs of your affected side may become stiff and tight because the neurotransmitters within the brain are failing to communicate to the muscle, tendon, and surrounding tissue. If spasticity is not treated, the muscles can freeze permanently into a tight fist, a bent elbow causing an arm to go to the chest, a stiff knee, a pointed foot (foot drop), and curled toes (hammer toes). Spasticity usually affects the joints of the elbow, wrist, knee, and ankle because the muscles tighten and bend the joint causing severe discomfort. Untreated spasticity can add considerable pain because of the abnormal positioning of the body.

Spasticity affects mobility. Mobility affects our socialization and leads to depression. It can become a vicious cycle of pain: staying in bed, getting bedsores, even contracting pneumonia. Severe spasticity can lead to nursing home care. Spasticity needs to be addressed.

What Is Shoulder Subluxation?

Also referred to as "joint instability," a subluxation is less than a dislocation. The shoulder joint surfaces may be compromised, but not dislocated. The ball of the upper arm joint has lost its bond with the shoulder socket due to spastic muscle contractions on the stroke-affected side. Subluxation pulls the arm bone into an abnormal position due to severe spasticity of the hemiplegic side (paralysis or partial-paralysis of one side of the body caused by stroke). The paralysis occurs on the side of the body opposite of where the stroke happened in the brain.

There is a great difference between shoulder pain after stroke and shoulder subluxation. If your affected arm just hung by your body after stroke and you didn't or couldn't move it for an extended period of time, you may have shoulder subluxation. The soft tissue within your arm and shoulder were strained and stretched by gravity. There are specialized arm slings available to aid in preventing and assisting those with shoulder subluxation. If you could move your affected arm a little more each day, but it may hurt to do so especially when you are tired, you have shoulder pain. In both cases, the muscles are weak.

97 The discomfort will begin to subside the more you are able to move your affected side. Sitting in one place for an extended period of time will worsen spasticity and shoulder pain. "Move it or lose it" is the old adage here.

98 Slow and steady progress will eventually lead to better movement. Use your other hand and arm to move your affected limb.

99 Ice packs alternating with heat for 10- to 15-minute intervals may relieve the pain.

100 Ibuprofen may be enough to relieve discomfort.

101 Meditation, gentle yoga, or swimming will help.

102 Range of motion exercises are imperative to prevent muscle weakening that can lead to shoulder pain, spasticity, or shoulder subluxation. Continuing a low-impact regular exercise program will lessen muscle spasms and help joints move.

103 When in bed, prop your arm up on an extra pillow so that your wrist, elbow, and shoulder are parallel. This may relieve pressure on your shoulder and the muscles.

104 There are various medical treatments for spasticity such as intrathecal baclofen (ITB) therapy where a small pump is surgically implanted to supply medication to the spinal cord, oral medications such as muscle relaxers, and injections to block the nerves and help relieve spasms in the muscles. When taking medication be sure to continue moving those stiff and ridged muscles and joints. **Natural treatments** include stretching, mild physical exercise, gentle yoga, and braces. The last resort to help your spasticity is surgery. Your physician will determine which treatment is right for you.

105 Technological appliances available today help prevent foot drop and address concerns regarding spasticity. Bioness is one company that works with spasticity issues. Saebo is another company that offers the Saebo Glove and Saebo Flex—Saebo Reach technology system.

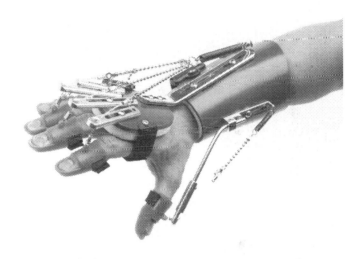

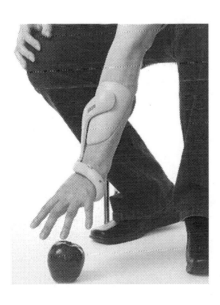

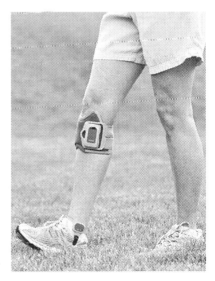

Central Nerve Pain/Thalamic Pain (Tips 106 and 107)

What Is Central Nerve Pain or Thalamic Pain?

If an ischemic stroke affects the thalamic region in the brain, a stroke survivor may experience sensations on the affected side of the body called "central nerve pain" (CNP) or "thalamic pain."

It may feel like a constant tingling or an icy sensation throughout the entire stroke-affected side, down to the bone, yet the stroke survivor may be unable to feel textures, water, hot or cold, or scratches, bumps, cuts, or bruises on the outside of the affected side. This is caused by the brain sending confused messages to the affected side of the body due to the stroke. The thalamus is the brain's "relay station" interpreting signals from one area of the brain to another.

There are many names for this post-stroke pain such as: "central post-stroke pain" (CPSP), "central pain syndrome" (CPS), "CPSP syndrome," or "posterior thalamic syndrome."

Central pain often begins shortly after stroke, but may be delayed by months or even years. When we have pain we want immediate relief, but that's not always possible. First, your physician will attempt to discover the reason for the pain. Is it muscle or joint pain associated with spasticity or shoulder subluxation or is it CPS? Next, your physician may try muscle relaxer medication along with mild exercise, possibly therapy, and comfort measures for relief before trying other measures. Central pain is coming directly from deep within the brain due to scrambled messages. The relay station is confused and sends incorrect information to the cerebral cortex.

106 Your neurologist or physician may prescribe medication to help manage the discomfort, recommend physical therapy, give injections of cortisone (steroids), or prescribe a transcutaneous electrical nerve stimulation (TENS) unit for you. TENS applies a small electrical current to the skin to promote muscle tone and help reduce pain. Also, your physician may refer you to a Pain Management unit or center.

107 There are things you can do at home to reduce pain from CNP too. Exercise by rolling the shoulders, stretching gently, walking, applying heat, or using various relaxation techniques.

Comfort Measures (Tips 108–124)

After a stroke, it may be difficult to position yourself because your stroke-affected side may not move as well. You may feel as if you are falling because sensory input is not functioning correctly.

What Is Sensory Input?

Stroke survivors are continually practicing this method during everyday living, possibly unaware of the medical term. By continually stimulating all five senses: touch, sight, hearing, speaking, and smell to evoke a response on your stroke-affected side, you are providing sensory input. Also, sensory input is important to our balance, movement, and coordination.

108 At night, a large body pillow stationed against your back with a smaller pillow between your knees may alleviate discomfort.

109 To improve sensory input, lie on your stroke-affected side for a very short time (10–15 seconds) every night. Then, roll onto your back for relief. At first, this exercise may be uncomfortable. By lengthening the time spent lying on your affected side, you will increase your tolerance and soon begin to feel new sensations throughout the affected body parts. Over time, your body will adjust and you may not feel as if you are going to fall when reclining on your stroke-affected side.

110 You may find that you want to protect your stroke-affected side by holding or cradling your affected arm with your unaffected hand—this is good for sensory input. Take it a step further and touch every part of your affected side. Knead your affected fingers and hand with your unaffected hand when you're watching television or relaxing in a chair. If you wear a brace on your affected arm, feel your affected fingers and try to bend them or wiggle them with your unaffected fingers. Try to move your affected fingers on their own. Even if they move a fraction of an inch, that's progress.

111 Touching material of various textures with your affected hand stimulates your brain. Lace your unaffected fingers between your affected fingers and place the palm and fingers of your affected hand on various fabrics and surfaces. This may feel very strange at first, but you are rewiring brain pathways as well as becoming aware of spatial fields on your affected side.

112 Use pressure sensitive putty or hand exercisers to improve strength and flexibility in your affected hand. These can be obtained through medical supply companies.

113 Scents can assist sensory input as well by producing a calm feeling.

114 Aromatherapy diffusers may be used to create relaxation. Check with your physician regarding the medication you are taking and the use of essential oils (oils from plants used for healing) as some oils may produce side effects with blood pressure medications, seizure medications, or antidepressants, for example. Ask your physician which type of aromatherapy diffuser (ultrasonic, evaporative, nebulizing, or heat) is right for you.

115 Use body lotion that has eucalyptus (a scent that clears the mind) and spearmint (an uplifting aroma). Rub the lotion into your hands (yes, both hands) before going to bed at night. Breathe in the relaxing aroma.

116 **Accumulate scents for sachets**. You will be getting out, walking, bending, gathering, and smelling. Make sachets of various outdoor scents you enjoy by placing a small amount of the fragrant material into a mesh bag. These can be refilled with different scents when the aroma wears out.

117 **Bring the scent of flowers indoors by cutting some of your own flowers or purchasing some**. You can even cut thorn roses if you're careful. Use a hand shears to clip the flowers then pick them up from the ground. If bending is difficult for you, use a reacher. (A reacher can be obtained through North Coast Functional Solutions catalog or medical supply stores.)

118 **Avoid candles**. Candles come in various scents, but if you have memory difficulties they are not a good choice.

119 **Use fragrances or spices in a potpourri pot**. Purchase an electric potpourri that shuts off automatically. In a small amount of water, simmer the comforting herbs and flavorings found in your spice rack, like cinnamon sticks, lemon, or vanilla.

120 **Many inexpensive aromatherapy diffusers are available and work well for a short time**. These contain a variety of scents in a small bottle and are sold with bamboo sticks. Place the bamboo sticks into the liquid to diffuse the aroma.

121 **Avoid spray air fresheners**. They contain various chemicals and the aroma doesn't last very long.

122 **A massage given by a massage therapist, or even your partner/spouse, improves sensory input and may enhance relaxation**.

123 Pressure point therapy or acupuncture is another alternative to enhancing sensory input or feedback. However, this treatment should be performed by a specialized therapist, with your physician's approval and recommendation.

124 Baths in Epsom salts relieve muscle strain and promote relaxation.

Activities of Daily Living (Tips 125–177)

Personal Care (Tips 125–126)

At first, you will find that personal care at home seems awkward when performing tasks one handed. We may not be acknowledging our stroke-affected side, but we do have two halves to our body. It may take longer to accomplish personal care than before the stroke. In time, and with a few helpful hints, the task will become easier and more familiar to you.

125 **Plan your actions before attempting a new task**. Take time to think about performing familiar tasks in a new way, and discover what works best for you.

126 **Do one task at a time**. For example, get the toothbrush out. Now, what goes with the toothbrush? Toothpaste. Get the toothpaste ready. Although this sounds easy, the task can be overwhelming within the first year post-stroke. It can be a struggle to think coherently and quickly.

Bathing or Showering
(Tips 127−140)

It is much safer to take a shower than to lower yourself into a slippery bathtub. It is also more difficult for a family member to assist you out of the tub. Here are some safety procedures and tips for each type of bathing.

127 **Add a handheld shower nozzle.** They are relatively inexpensive and easy to install. A handheld shower nozzle will be helpful in rinsing your hair and body without the necessity of turning around in the shower to do so.

128 **Install grab bars in your shower or bath.** The types that securely screw into the wall are better than the types that hold by suction alone.

129 **Place a large nonskid bathmat in your shower or tub.**

130 **Plastic pump bottles attached to the wall or hung from a shower caddy are easier to use with one hand.** Shampoo, liquid soap, lotions, or anything you use in the shower or directly afterwards should be in plastic containers to prevent breakage.

131 **A wash mitt or nylon puff is easier to manage than a washcloth.**

132 **An elongated scrubber with loops at both ends (for grasping) works best for washing your back.** These types of scrubbers have terry cloth on one side and a rougher texture on the other side. Loop it over your affected fingers, placing the loop between your thumb and palm, place the scrubber over your shoulder, and grasp it with your unaffected hand. This technique also works well for moving your stroke-affected arm and hand.

133 A short-handled dish-washing sponge works well for washing your stroke-affected side.

134 Have everything close at hand. Gather the soap, wash mitt, shampoo, conditioner, long-handled brush, sponges, mesh puffs, scrubbers, lotion, towels, and anything else you will need prior to entering the shower or tub.

135 A tub bench may be easier. Medical supply company catalogs, such as from North Coast Functional Solutions, sell shower or tub seats that attach to the side of the tub.

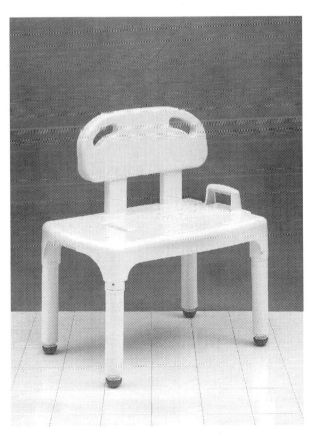

136 Test the water temperature with your unaffected hand prior to getting into the shower or tub.

137 Use care getting into the tub. Sit on the edge of the tub and place your unaffected foot in the tub first; then use a wall-attached grab bar to hold on to and lower yourself carefully into the tub.

138 Exercise your affected shoulder, arm, and hand during bathing. While seated safely in the shower or tub, try rolling your shoulders in circles. One shoulder at a time or together. Scrunch up your shoulders until they are as close to your ears as possible. Release the shoulders and let them drop. Turn your head to look over one shoulder, then slowly forward, then to the other shoulder. Next, hold your stroke-affected hand with your other hand and gently guide your affected arm out in front of you as much as possible. While holding your stroke-affected hand, try raising your hands in the air as high as possible. If there is pain, back off, as bath time is supposed to be a relaxing, pleasurable experience. Knead your affected fingers with your other hand. You are providing crucial data to your brain during bath time stretches too.

139 Use care getting out of the tub. To avoid slipping while getting out of the tub, let the water drain out. Dry yourself in the tub. Place a towel on the drained surface of the tub. Reach for the grab bar, bend your legs, plant your feet, and stand up. Sit on the side of the tub and swing one leg at a time out of the tub. As long as the bathroom stays warm and you don't get chilled, this technique may work for you.

140 Applying body lotion after your bath helps you observe body parts for pressure, swelling, or redness. If you are diabetic, this is a good time to check your feet for sores, pitted swelling, or discoloration. Make sure you rub lotion into your stroke-affected hand too. Again, this is a time to move as much of the hand as possible by using your other hand for support and guidance. Even though there may be no sensation in your affected hand, moving it as much as possible will improve circulation, recognition, and movement.

Dressing and Undressing (Tips 141–153)

You have known how to dress yourself ever since you were a child. Why is the task so difficult after a stroke? A very simplified answer to a complex situation that has occurred within the brain is that the stroke-affected area in the brain may be short circuiting some connections. But let's move on to performing some of these basic skills once again.

141 **Before going to bed at night, lay out all the clothing you will wear the next day.** Underwear and socks should go on the top of the pile as you will put them on first. Next, the outer clothing: shirt/blouse, pants, and shoes.

142 **Dress and undress in a sitting position as much as possible.** It will be easier, and much safer.

143 **Undress your unaffected side first and clothe your affected side first.**

144 **Establish a routine of getting dressed every day.** These repetitive steps will not only boost neuroplasticity within your brain, but help you emotionally as well.

145 **Women may want to consider a different type of brassiere.** Front closure or stretchy sports bras may be easier to put on than regular back closure bras. If you have a back closure bra, you can hook it closed by putting it on backwards. Then, turn it around on your body and place your affected arm into the bra strap, followed by the other arm; bend forward and lift each strap up individually. In removing the bra, use the opposite procedure. Slide the strap off the unaffected shoulder and slip your arm out. Then slip your arm out of the strap of your affected side. Turn the bra around and unhook the clasp.

146 **T-shirts or shirts that fit over the head are easier to manage than shirts with buttons.**

147 **Women who have a stroke-affected left side may want to consider wearing men's shirts that have large buttons as they close in the opposite direction.**

148 **Shirts that button at the wrist should be tried on before purchasing because they are extremely difficult to button one handed.** Make sure the wristband is large enough for your hand to fit through with the button closed.

149 **Blouses or shirts with small buttons can be slipped over your head** with only one or two buttons unfastened, as if it were a tee shirt, and then the buttons can be fastened. The blouse or shirt must be large enough to accommodate putting the garment on your affected arm first, pulling it up on the arm to elbow length, placing your unaffected arm in the sleeve in the same manner, and slipping it over your head and down your body.

150 **Keep it simple when it comes to clothing.** And simple doesn't mean it can't be stylish. It is much better to wear clothing you can manage alone than wearing clothing that you may need help with for dressing or toileting.

151 **Shoes that have a sturdy thick rubber sole and come up high on your instep stay on your stroke-affected foot better than other types.** Some of these styles include sports shoes, shoes with zip closures on the instep, bear claw sandals, pull-on style boots, or walking shoes that can be laced with self-closure type laces. If you have an ankle-foot orthotic (AFO), your therapist may recommend a specific shoe for you.

Ladies, comfortable supportive shoes are more important to safety and movement than high heels are to fashion. Avoid a trip to the emergency room because of a broken ankle caused by wearing high heels.

152 **Consider purchasing two pairs of shoes for the price of one by checking with shoe outlet stores or online.** Your AFO may require a size larger than your other foot wears. When you purchase shoes, you may have to buy two pairs in order to compensate for the brace.

153 **Mittens or gloves are the options during winter.** Whatever you choose, keep your fingers and hands covered in the cold. You may not feel your fingers post-stroke, but they're still subject to frostbite. If you live in a cold part of the country where winters are harsh, the snow is deep, and the layered look is protocol, mittens may be easier to manage, at least for the first year post-stroke. Some stroke survivors will opt to wear a mitten on their affected hand and a glove on their unaffected hand. If you choose to wear mittens, make sure the cuff pulls up far enough to stay on your affected hand. If you choose to wear gloves, try purchasing a pair that is a size larger than you normally wear. Look for a pair that has a wrist strap that can be tightened or loosened to keep the glove on your hand.

During my first winter post-stroke, I wore mittens, but during the spring, summer, and fall, I worked toward putting a glove on my affected hand. I can't feel my fingers, especially when they're inside the glove where I can't see them, so I have to fish for each finger to work it into the glove. This takes time, patience, practice, and determination.

Nail Care (Tips 154–158)

154 **If you are diabetic, consult your physician regarding your specific foot care procedures.**

155 Check fingernails and toenails on your affected side frequently. Throw embarrassment out the window when it comes to getting help to clip the toenails or fingernails on your affected side. If you are having difficulty bending or reaching or have vision or balance issues, your nails still have to be maintained so that shoes do not injure your feet and fingernails don't accidently scratch yourself or others.

156 Try filing fingernails on your unaffected hand using this home remedy. Ask a friend, neighbor, or relative with carpentry skills to cut a groove, small enough to hold an emery board, into a block of well-sanded wood. Place an emery board securely into the groove. Then, you may be able to file your nails. (This grooved block of wood works great for playing cards as well.)

157 Pamper yourself and get a professional manicure and pedicure. Not only does this professional service solve the difficulty associated with nail care but it provides other opportunities as well. By getting out of the house, you are building self-esteem, stimulating plasticity by making the appointment and travel arrangements, and communicating with others. If your affected hand is difficult to control during a manicure, hold the fingers on the table with your unaffected hand. There is a lot of brain work involved in this tip. But you will be rewarded with more than pretty nails.

158 Nail care is a great time to notice and manipulate your stroke-affected hand and foot.

Shaving (Tips 159–168)

There are many ways to remove hair from unwanted areas. You can use an electric razor, a disposable razor, depilatory hair removal products such as creams, or go to a professional salon for waxing or sugaring (the sugar technique uses natural ingredients and is better for sensitive skin), or use a laser hair-removal system.

159 **For ease and safety, consider using an electric shaver after a stroke.** However, blades or razor heads may have to be changed frequently. If an electric razor feels too intense for your stroke-affected side, consider an alternative.

160 **Inexpensive disposable safety razors might be for you, as you don't have to worry about changing blades.**

161 **Men can apply shaving cream or foam to the back of their affected hand and use their other hand to apply the cream to their face.**

162 **Be very careful shaving stroke-affected areas,** because you may easily cut places that lack sensation.

163 **Use a large mirror and provide good lighting.** You may have visual difficulties post-stroke and not be aware of one side of your body, including your face, and for women, legs and underarms. Turn your head slowly from left to right to help improve any visual difficulties you may be experiencing. Use your unaffected fingers to feel for unshaven areas on your affected side. (More about mirrors in Chapter 7, tips 390–393)

Women

164 **When shaving your stroke-affected underarm,** lean forward and let your affected arm dangle away from your body— then reach in to shave.

165 **Another technique** is to lift your affected bicep parallel with your shoulder and let your forearm and hand relax.

Shave under the arm. Both techniques require practice. This one requires the ability to move your stroke-affected arm.

166 **Shaving your unaffected armpit will present more of a challenge**. This is where duct tape and a tongue depressor or dowel come into play. Tape the tongue depressor (pick up a few at your local pharmacy) or dowel to the handle of the razor to extend it as far as is comfortable for you to reach your armpit with your unaffected hand. Eventually, your stroke-affected hand may become coordinated enough to hold the razor and participate in this task.

167 **Shaving your legs can be done while you are seated in the bathtub**. Use shaving cream and shave with your unaffected hand. Be careful if you prop up your affected leg while in the bathtub.

168 **An alternative** is to sit in a chair and prop your affected leg up on another chair while you shave your leg.

Hair Care (Tips 169–171)

169 **A short hairstyle** that can easily be maintained is most practical during stroke recovery.

170 **Use a wall-mounted hairdryer**, so you can style your hair while drying it.

171 **If you have long hair,** use a claw clip, banana clip, or hair band to keep your hair in place.

Dental Care (Tips 172–177)

172 **Try not to use your teeth to compensate for your stroke-affected limb.** After a stroke, you may be tempted to use your teeth to assist you, rather than using your affected hand. Dental work is expensive. Some things should not be placed in your mouth. Most importantly, you will be forming negative adaptability practices instead of stimulating your affected side.

173 **Attend regular dental appointments and alert your dentist to all medications you are taking, prior to teeth cleaning or dental surgery.**

174 **An electric ultrasonic toothbrush** works well for teeth cleaning, tartar control, and gum stimulation.

175 **A long-handled disposable flossing pick** can be easily used after brushing to remove food particles and prevent gum disease.

176 **Apply a small amount of toothpaste to the back of your stroke-affected hand and wipe it off with the toothbrush.** Voila! The toothpaste and toothbrush are united and ready to be used. You recognized and used your stroke-affected arm and hand as well.

177 **If you have dentures or a partial dental plate**, after soaking in a dental cleaning solution, rinse thoroughly, apply adhesive if needed, and insert the denture or partial plate using your unaffected hand.

Taking the Sting Out of Stroke (Tips 178–192)

Self-Esteem (Tips 178–184)

This chapter addresses a philosophy of stroke recovery that will hopefully help you by taking the sting out of stroke and replacing it with more powerful images.

There is a gift within each of us that is more dominant than the effects stroke may have left on our bodies or minds. It is that spark within you. Some people may call it your "soul," your "spirit," or your "being," but everyone was born with this precious quality. This force is called upon to give us courage, comfort, and strength.

178 **Our power lies in our reaction to our daily challenges**. Stroke is an adversity that changes our direction, and even greater—our bodies and minds. It is the dichotomy of our spirit that says, "life isn't fair," but at the same time empowers us to embrace life.

179 **It takes time to learn about your particular medical condition**. You begin to process information as a chemist does in a lab, slowly and carefully. Learn all you can about your particular stroke. Become your own best advocate. But first give yourself the gift of time to allow yourself to recover to the best of your ability.

180 **Aspects of stroke recovery are ongoing in different forms as we slowly learn to adapt**. Hospital physical therapy is replaced by our firm commitment to continue daily exercise and learn how to perform our daily tasks in a new way while at home. Vocational and occupational therapy are transformed into our reaching out to our community resources, like Rehabilitation Services in helping us devise new ways of accomplishing our goals. Recreational therapy morphs into fun activities like hobbies and community involvement. Finally, neuropsychological therapy changes into family intervention needed to understand our personal stroke story to continue on a better path in the world around us.

181 **Among the many challenges we face come opportunities for personal, educational, and spiritual growth**. For example, there may be an opportunity to enhance a hobby or special interest by visiting your local rehabilitation service or by using the Ticket to Work program offered by your local Social Security office. There are also opportunities to learn. You may have the opportunity to go to college or take a community educational course. An opportunity for spiritual or religious growth happens quickly when we face medical and emotional challenges. Seek a spiritual leader of your religious affiliation for advice and direction.

182 **You may need to call upon new strategies and innovative skills**. Be patient with yourself, keep a healing journal, and focus on one goal at a time.

183 **Family dynamics require understanding**. Find the balance between your family's time constraints and independence of each family member. Slow down and modify your lifestyle to involve problem solving.

184 **A safe environment is priority for all people healing from the effects of stroke.** The most important aspect of our environment is feeling safe around the people we love, respect, and rely on to help us heal. If there is ever an issue with your safety, call 911 immediately.

The Healing Power of Humor (Tips 185–192)

Sometimes, stroke survivors understand only literal meanings or concrete language and cannot understand jokes that others "get." A stroke survivor may have difficulty interpreting abstract language like metaphors, inferences, and nonverbal cues. Because of the stroke, problems may arise in following the rules of communication by saying inappropriate things, not using facial expressions, talking at the wrong time, or becoming extremely talkative.

Pseudobulbar affect (PBA) or emotional lability should not be confused with a lack of insight. PBA is an involuntary action.

A quick description of what is going on in the brain to cause this difficulty is necessary. When a stroke affects the right hemisphere of the brain, causing weakness on the left part of the body, a stroke survivor may not be aware of complications regarding social communication or insight. The cognitive processes (thinking, understanding, learning, and remembering) may be disrupted.

This stroke side effect should not be confused with Alzheimer's disease, dementia, or the popular term "senior moments," even though a stroke survivor may be having difficulty recalling information like the date, time, birth dates, age, or familiar names. Within stroke, it is a problem with orientation. In time, this difficulty may improve.

Slowly, we relearn to make the jump from what is considered inappropriate to appropriate language and humor. We begin to smile when it comes to our own foibles.

185 **The humor of what we do while healing from stroke may be lost until we are ready and able to heal from the inside out**. Carol Burnet said, "Comedy is tragedy plus time." Stroke is certainly a tragedy.

That inside place for humor may be spontaneously awakened by watching your favorite standup comedian, or viewing a humorous cartoon, or merely observing the daily rituals of those around you. When you think of it, the new way you learned to dress after stroke may put a smile on your face. For women, putting a bra on backwards doesn't seem natural. But I soon realized that my 18-hour bra lived up to its name because it took me about that long to learn to put it on!

186 **Use humor as your arsenal in the fight toward healing**. Humor can be found in the most unlikely places and spaces in our lives. As recovery progresses, we begin to understand the meaning of figurative speech.

187 **When you purposefully laugh, it means that the grieving process is making way for the healing to begin**. When you are able to laugh at something you said that you didn't actually mean to say, you are learning to flip the tragedy of stroke into humor.

188 **Humor can be very complicated**. Certainly we don't want the public to perceive stroke survivors as comedians or laugh at issues of disability. But to suddenly understand humor is an extremely important milestone to pass on the road to recovery. Our brain is finally able to make that leap from concrete to abstract thinking. Wow! Those brain cells are connecting—we "get it!"

189 **Language is more than the words; it is the tone, pace, expression, and innuendoes that also make up communication**. Timing and synchronization is vital to recovering all of our senses, including our sense of humor.

190 **We are resilient**. When you are able to comprehend humor, you are unconsciously reconnecting brain synapses and neurotransmitters. When you are able to purposefully laugh, you are on the right path.

191 **Practice smiling**. Others will wonder what you're up to.

192 **Further resources on our brain's capacity to interpret humor** can be found at www.oliversacks.com, the website of the late Oliver Sacks, a renowned neurologist and former professor at the New York University (NYU) School of Medicine. He authored many books, including *The Man Who Mistook His Wife for a Hat*.

Another resource is the Association for Applied and Therapeutic Humor (AATH; www.aath.org), a nonprofit, international community of humor and laughter professionals and advocates. In 1987, Alison L. Crane, RN, established the AATH to provide education, resources, and support by promoting "therapeutic humor." As the website explains, therapeutic humor stimulates health and wellness by inspiring "a playful appreciation of the incongruity of life's situations." This organization enhances health practices and helps people work toward physical, emotional, cognitive, social, and spiritual healing. As an author and professional speaker, I have presented "The No Joke Stroke— How Humor Helps Heal" at an annual convention of the AATH.

Because this information relates specifically to the topic of humor, it is given here, as a tip for further reading, rather than in the resource section.

Nutrition
(Tips 193–216)

Dysphagia (Tips 193–198)

A swallowing difficulty following stroke is called "dysphagia." Sometimes, stroke survivors may be unaware of having dysphagia or the symptoms associated with it. They just begin to choke on food or liquids that they never had a problem consuming before the stroke.

Let's sidetrack to medical definitions to clarify a couple of terms. In medical terminology, the prefix "a" means an absence while the prefix "dys" means abnormal. Therefore, "dysphagia" means abnormal swallowing.

On the other hand, "dysphasia," with an "s" instead of a "g," refers to a language disorder or abnormality in the ability to speak, read, write, or comprehend. When the condition is moderate, without total speech disruption, it is called dysphasia. When one or all of these symptoms become severe to the point of total loss of speech, the word "aphasia" is used.

193 If you notice any inability to swallow or you begin to choke or gag on food or liquids once you are home after having a stroke, contact your physician immediately. However, most dysphagia difficulties post-stroke will have been discovered by your physician or therapist while you were in the hospital.

194 **Tuck your chin toward your chest when swallowing to prevent choking**.

195 **Liquids may need to be thickened with an additive** prescribed by your physician or physiatrist, a doctor of physical medicine and rehabilitation (PM&R), to assist you when swallowing.

196 **Soft foods or foods processed in a blender may be easier to swallow** without choking than bite-size pieces of food.

197 **Chew food on the unaffected side of your mouth**.

198 **Check for trapped food in the affected side of your mouth**.

Mealtimes (Tips 199–200)

There's a lot to process within the brain while eating: preparing small bites of food, placing the food on a fork or spoon, chewing, and swallowing. Distractions caused by eating in a noisy restaurant or surrounded by lively table conversation may precipitate problems with chewing or swallowing food properly and lead to occasional choking for any stroke survivor.

199 **Mealtime should be a quiet time**. Don't worry about answering questions, carrying on table conversation, or listening while you are eating. One activity at a time is appropriate after stroke.

200 Take very small bites of food. Rushing through a meal is unnecessary, especially after stroke.

Nutrition (Tips 201–216)

Nutrition addresses lifelong goals toward balanced meals for stroke survivors. We need to know what foods carry high-risk factors for stroke, as well as foods that keep our hearts and arteries healthy as we reap the benefits of increasing energy and metabolism.

201 Anything you take into your body affects the brain. Whether it is prescribed medications, over-the-counter medications, foods, liquids, illegal drugs, legal or illegal marijuana, or tobacco products; and no matter the means whether orally, intravenously, inhaling, and so forth—if it gets into the blood stream, it gets into the brain.

Some things are good for us and are meant to alter our brain or blood chemistry, such as prescribed medication. Others are not good and will deter stroke recovery or even predetermine our ultimate outcome. What are you doing to your body to help it function properly and become strong? This very important question involves everything you put into your frame to build a healthy body, mind, and spirit.

202 Keep those brain cells healthy by staying hydrated. We need water to loosen constricted muscles. We need water for our brain to function properly. We need water to dilute medications we may be taking. Water will plump up our blood vessels and help circulation. We need at least 64 ounces of water per day. If you drink half the amount of water in the morning and the other half in the afternoon, you could have this daily requirement completed by 8 p.m. so you may not have to get up during the night to use the toilet. Water is free and the best resource we have toward healthy living.

203 **Reduce your alcohol use**. Alcohol is a depressant. Stroke survivors don't need to increase a feeling of depression.

204 **Add fresh fruits to your daily nutrition**. The old adage, "An apple a day keeps the doctor away" isn't far from the truth. We need this fast-burning type of natural sugar that breaks down quickly in our bodies. Bananas contain potassium which helps decrease muscle cramps.

205 **Avoid dark green vegetables, like broccoli, if you are taking a prescribed blood-thinning medication**. There is a side effect associated with eating dark green vegetables while on blood thinners: the medication may cause bleeding.

Most vegetables can be eaten raw after washing, or steamed, or added to your favorite recipe. Try vegetables and fruits that you haven't tried in the past; perhaps you will acquire a taste for something different. Sensory input can change the way foods taste as well.

206 **Avoid the deli department except for rare occasions**. The foods in the deli are already prepared—so fast and convenient, but not necessarily nutritious. Most of the side dishes at a deli contain mayonnaise or are high in fat and oils that are not easily broken down by our bodies but stored as fat and cholesterol. Avoid cholesterol.

207 **Avoid fast food places as much as possible**—we're searching for brain- and body-building fuel.

208 **Buy skinless, boneless chicken because cholesterol is contained in the skin**.

209 **Sodium is not our friend**. Avoid eating processed foods, especially cold cuts or prepacked lunch meats, wieners, sausages, and bacon, or anything processed in a high concentration of salt. If you must have bacon, try turkey bacon but only occasionally.

210 **Purchase fresh or frozen fish** without breading. Meat is fine occasionally. The body can't break down fibrous meat as effectively as soft, flaky, fish. Meat can also be a choking hazard with some stroke survivors.

211 **Stay away from anything made with white flour.** White bread products are high in calories and low in nutritional value. Buy whole grain bread (whole wheat bread is not the same as whole grain). Also, brown rice and whole grain pasta is better for you than the alternative white. Most stroke survivors are not as active as before the stroke. If we consume foods high in calories without having the body use food, we will gain weight. Extra weight can be dangerous for stroke survivors.

212 **Watch out for the sugar content in cold cereals.** Sugar adds to obesity issues. Sugar wreaks havoc on those with diabetes or those who might be at risk. Hot cereal such as oatmeal and cream of wheat are better choices.

213 **Juices that contain 100% pure juice are good choices** as others may contain added sugar. Stroke survivors need to avoid refined sugar (glucose) especially when diabetic.

214 **Setting specific meal times may assist memory and help the body recover.** "Did I eat today? What did I eat? I can't remember." If this sounds familiar to you, setting specific times to eat may be an option. Sometimes, by forgetting when or what we have eaten, we begin to feed an emotional need instead of a bodily need. This can lead to obesity.

215 **Have someone go food shopping with you until you feel comfortable doing it alone.** Nutritional choices can be difficult within the first year or so post-stroke. Logical thinking patterns may be disrupted. Making appropriate choices, while listening to others and music in the background, can overwhelm sensory input and produce stress.

After shopping for food, it's time to rest. Shopping requires exercise—walking or using a motorized cart, bending, reaching, stretching, reading, comprehension, making choices, and communication. You did it! You may be exhausted but consider this; could you have completed this task when you first came home from rehabilitation?

2.16 **Another alternative is delivery service meals**. There are about 13 companies in the United States that provide healthy meals through delivery service. This makes food shopping easier, but you will be required to prepare the meals after delivery. These "dinner in a box" options can be expensive, but they provide healthier choices than other call-in or order-on-line options like sandwiches or pizza. Eat healthy food any way that is convenient and cost effective for you as you recover.

Around the House (Tips 217–279)

Cooking (Tips 217–233)

Now that we've completed purchasing the food, we have to prepare it. If we clean up as we go it won't be as difficult. So let's get started.

217 Use a stainless steel, spiked cutting board with a vise grip to hold food while cutting.

218 Place newspaper on prep areas and under your cutting board for easier clean up. I challenge anyone to prepare a meal one handed (hemiparesis is weakness on one side of the body) while feeling as if they have blinders on (visual difficulties) without making a mess!

219 When using a recipe, gather all the needed ingredients first. Then, place a pencil mark on the recipe after adding the ingredient or completing the step. This process may help you remember what you've done and what to do next.

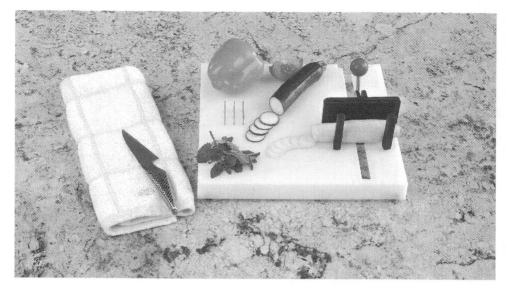

Swedish cutting board with vise grips, available
through North Coast Functional Solutions catalog.

220 **Peel carrots, potatoes, or any vegetable by first securing
them on the cutting board spikes.** Make sure the suction
cups are secured to the counter for a firm grip.

221 **Use a food processor**—slicing and dicing may be accomplished using an easier method.

222 **Make sure your knives are sharp and your affected hand
and fingers are well out of the way.** A wall-mounted knife
sharpener works well for one-handed sharpening.

223 **Avoid trying to carry hot or bulky items to or from the
stove!** If using a large cooking pot, fill a smaller pitcher or
measuring cup with the liquid needed and pour it into the
pot on the range top.

224 **There are a few ways to anchor a bowl or pan to prevent it
from spinning around while stirring or mixing one handed.**
(1) Use a suction cup sticky bowl appliance that fastens to
your counter and the bottom of the bowl (check the North

Coast Functional Solutions catalog). (2) Sit on a chair and place the mixing bowl between your thighs. (3) Place the mixing bowl in a kitchen drawer, close the drawer around the bowl to secure it, apply pressure with your body weight if necessary, and mix the ingredients. Stirring on the stovetop can be managed by anchoring the pan handle counterclockwise against another heavier pan placed on the back burner while stirring clockwise in the pan placed on the front burner ballast.

225 **To place or remove items from the oven, use a long, padded oven mitt. If the item is too heavy to lift with your unaffected hand, ask for assistance.**

226 **Microwave ovens located above a range-top cooking surface are dangerous post-stroke.** Microwaves provide fast and efficient food preparation. However, lifting hot items out of a microwave when stretching upwards one handed with visual difficulties is hazardous.

227 **Opening a can requires a can opener that you can operate with one hand.** If you use a hand crank can opener, pierce the can with the opener using your unaffected hand. Then switch hands and stabilize the opener with whatever grip you have with your affected hand and turn the crank with your unaffected hand and fingers. This is exercise for both hands, because as one hand turns the crank, the affected hand is holding the two handles closed. It may be difficult at first, but you will be learning to use both hands.

228 **A cordless handheld opener is another option.** Check stores, online, or adaptability catalogues to see which can opener works best for you.

229 **Opening jars can be difficult.** Place the jar between your thighs when you are sitting and place a rubber mat over the lid or a thick rubber band around the seal of the lid. Hold the jar in place by gripping your thighs together as much as possible and twist on the rubber mat or rubber band using your unaffected hand. This procedure can be used to break the seal and open plastic caps on bottles or other containers too.

230 **A pair of adaptable large-handled kitchen scissors is useful for various kitchen tasks,** for example, opening plastic bags or other items purchased at stores. (Check North Coast Functional Solutions catalog online or your area's adaptability supply store.)

231 **When setting the table, use nonbreakable dishes, cups, and glasses. Keep a simple caddy on the table at all times**. It keeps napkins, silverware, and condiments easily accessible. These types of containers can be found in houseware departments or online.

232 **Plastic containers with seal tight lids or zipper type storage bags work well for refrigerator food storage**. To remove the air from a zip-type bag, place the bag on the counter and roll the bag until the air is released. Hold the bag securely with your affected arm and zip the bag with your unaffected hand.

233 **Food that is sold precut, in individual servings, or as a fresh package meal may be more convenient and easier to prepare**. Vegetables, salads, chicken, seafood fillets, all-in-one stews and stir-fries are a few examples. Eat nutritiously while conserving energy.

Cleaning (Tips 234–259)

Not very many people enjoy doing housework but it has to be done. So let's get started.

234 **Forget about being a perfectionist**. We want our environment clean and items put away so it doesn't cause confusion and stress.

Laundry

If your washer and dryer are located in the basement, beware, because there's a terrible hazard between you and the appliances—the stairs. There may be exposed cement at the bottom of the stairs and even if there is carpeting, it may not prevent serious complications from a fall.

235 **Laundry isn't as important as you are**. There can be several steep and narrow steps between you and the appliances. Your therapist will instruct you on the proper technique for climbing up and stepping down stairways. Attempting stairs before you are ready is disastrous.

236 **Never use the stairs without someone to assist you**.

237 **Never venture down a flight of stairs without a cell phone/smartphone or cordless phone in your pocket to call for help if necessary**.

Let's assume you reached the washer and dryer on the main level of your home.

238 **You can use one hand to sort the clothes, if necessary, and afterwards operate your washer and dryer**.

239 **Empty the clean clothes into a roller cart and push or pull it to a chair. Sit down to fold the clothes**.

240 **Smaller items are easier to fold than larger ones, but don't get discouraged**. Someone can always help you do the folding sheet dance and you can use your unaffected hand and your opposing elbow and body to assist you with this partnered two step.

241 **Match socks, then fold the pair in half**. This is a great way to increase visual field by turning your head, and increase sensory input by size, shape, and feel of texture. Increase memory by finding the mate-less sock.

242 **Do the best you can with folding and distributing laundry**. Place the folded laundry in the wheeled cart and push it from room to room, placing the clothes in their appropriate drawers or closets. You're working at stroke recovery as well by remembering where everything belongs. If you can't remember, don't fret. Leave the clothes in the appropriate room. If you can't remember rooms or how to match the clothes with the correct family member, sit down with your family and ask them to take their clothes out of the laundry cart. Even by observing, you are relearning.

243 **Use plastic or cloth-covered hangers**. The larger hangers are easier to grasp.

244 **Folding your pants**. Grab the bottom of both legs of the pants and shake the pants using your unaffected hand. If the pant legs are twisted, straighten them, repeat firm shake. Lay the pants on the table or a long flat surface. Using your unaffected hand, put the four seams of the pants together. Lay the bottom of the pants between the bottom and top of the hanger. Slide the hanger to the middle portion of the pants and pick up. Your pants are ready for the closet.

245 **Hanging your shirts**. Place the plastic hanger up from the body of the shirt to the neckline. For a blouse or shirt, button the top button while the shirt is lying on the table facing you. Place the hanger under the front closed button and up by the collar, hang the shirt or blouse up and adjust the shoulder seams on the hanger with your unaffected hand.

Polishing Furniture

246 **A long-handled lightweight magnetic duster works well for high places like drapery tops or ceiling fan blades**. Stroke survivors don't climb. We're inventive!

247 A dusting mitt works well for tables and low areas. Some come with treated fabric in the mitt for shining and polishing. This is a great range of motion exercise.

Vacuuming

248 A lightweight vacuum cleaner that you can handle is much easier than one you have to drag around. Let's avoid tripping over bulky objects.

249 A small handheld vacuum works great for little messes and they can be snapped into their recharging holder for easy access. They are easy to operate using one hand.

250 If you live with someone and a large clunky vacuum cleaner is the only option, trade the vacuuming for dusting or folding clothes.

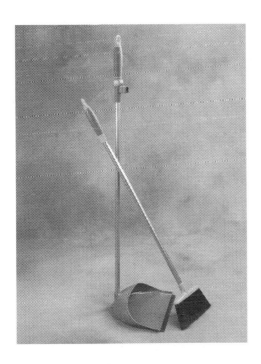

Sweeping the Kitchen or Bathroom Floor

251 Sweeping with one hand is easy if you position the broom handle across your unaffected shoulder and grab the broom lower down on the shaft. Better yet, purchase a long handle broom and dust pan from North Coast Functional Solutions catalog. The long-handled dust pan makes it much easier to keep you upright and steady while sweeping material into the pan.

252 You can use a lightweight portable vacuum, or the broom and dust pan described above, to sweep the kitchen and bathroom floors as well.

Cleaning the Floor

253 Use a floor steamer or all-in-one floor-cleaning system to avoid the traditional on-all-fours method of floor cleaning.

Making the Beds

254 Try making one side of the bed at a time as this saves steps. Do the bottom sheet, top sheet, and blanket or comforter before venturing to the other side of the bed.

255 Use a comforter as it's much easier to lay across the bed and doesn't require tucking in.

256 Sit down to replace pillow cases.

Washing and Drying Dishes

257 Use a dish drainer to anchor dishes and utensils in the sink while washing them with a long-handled scrubber. Then, rinse the dishes thoroughly and place them in another dish drainer in the adjacent sink. If you have a dishwasher, rinse the dishes and pans before loading.

258 **To help with memory difficulties, use a magnet on your dishwasher that flips to indicate whether your dishes are clean or dirty.** You may have used this little warning tag before the stroke too. (Why did we ignore this simple task prior to the stroke? You're not alone.)

Tips for Carrying Things (Tips 259–265)

259 **Wear a smock or hunting vest equipped with several pockets to carry lightweight objects.** Be careful not to overload the pockets or you may become unstable.

260 **Practice carrying an empty polyfoam cup in your affected hand and walking a few steps.** Gradually, work your way up to carrying an empty paper cup, an empty soda can, or another nonbreakable empty item.

261 **Practice carrying an empty nonbreakable plate and utensils in preparation for the dreaded buffet line.**

262 **When eating buffet style,** try to sit at a table close to the buffet. Avoid steps when attempting to carry and balance a plate of food. Fill your glass only halfway when carrying and carry it separately. Avoid trying to carry coffee or other hot items. Do what you are able to do and request assistance when needed.

263 Shoulder purses, back packs, or small pouches snapped together around your waist allow for hands-free carrying.

264 Reusable or recycled cloth bags are easier to carry, and stronger than grocery bags.

265 Purchase a folding push cart. This type of cart folds up for easy storage but expands to a deep, narrow basket for carrying groceries or other items. It is inexpensive and extremely handy for apartment dwellers too. You can also load the cart with laundry and detergent for trips to the laundry room.

Home Maintenance (Tips 266–279)

You've had a stroke but you may own a home. This requires keeping the equity up by performing home maintenance and seasonal chores.

266 Homeownership may allow a "disabled" person (stroke survivor) a discount on property tax in some states. Check with your accountant, tax preparer, or state property tax office for the proper qualifications and how to apply.

Even with decreased property taxes, you have the same responsibilities in maintenance and upkeep as any other homeowner. Spring and summer mandates mowing the grass, cleaning the pool, trimming and/or gardening. Autumn calls for leaf raking and cleaning rain gutters. In many parts of the nation, winter demands shoveling snow.

267 **Know your capabilities**. Planning each task is essential. Start gradually until you build endurance. Rest frequently and take your time. Slow and steady wins every time.

Summer

268 **If you have balance or coordination difficulties or are using an adaptive aid, hire someone to do the job for you.** Pushing, even a self-propelled lawn mower, can be exhausting after stroke.

269 **If you are able to tackle the job yourself,** a lightweight cordless electric lawnmower is easier than gas engine types. Mow in small sections, rest, and stay hydrated.

270 **Long-handled manual clippers are easier and safer to use for edging work versus an electric weed whacker.**

Autumn

271 **Raking leaves uses the same principle as sweeping the floor with a broom.** It can be done one handed by holding the rake with your unaffected hand and resting the handle against your shoulder. If you want to switch positions, use your stroke-affected hand and arm to stabilize the rake and pull with your unaffected hand. Rake the leaves onto a large tarp and gather the sides together and drag a small bundle at a time to your flowerbeds to cover them for the winter.

272 **Your lawn mower may have mulching capabilities.** This is another way to get rid of leaves in the fall, if the leaves are not too dense or wet. Again, if you are using an adaptive aid, hire someone or ask a family member to help you.

273 **Barter with neighbors**. You could agree to wash their car or wash a few reachable windows or provide a meal, for example, if they clean out your rain gutters. Climbing a ladder is not recommended for stroke survivors with one-sided weakness and/or coordination or mobility difficulties. Knowing your limits will prevent accidents and possibly build neighborly relations.

274 **There are a few alternatives for cleaning gutters**. A hose affixed to a gutter wand, attaching tools to a wet/dry shop vacuum, or a long-reaching pole to remove leaves while standing on the ground may work for cleaning gutters too. Although this tip and the next applies to everyone, it's nice to know stroke survivors are not alone.

275 **Hire a gutter cleaning company or handyman service to do this chore**. This might be the right choice for you. Check your area for services and prices.

276 **If a task is beyond your capability, ask for assistance**. There is more than one way to accomplish a task. What is the best and safest way to get a job done? You can ask for assistance but stay with your helper to watch and learn.

Winter

277 **Prepare ahead of time**. During late autumn, make a list of area snow-plowing services or neighbors who could shovel or use their snow blower to help you. Check what their prices are, how often they would help, and when they expect payment. Some areas offer volunteer services as well. This better prepares you for unexpected snow storms and relieves stress.

278 **Try to keep ahead of the heavy snow by shoveling often if you decide to go it alone**. Snow shoveling can be difficult for anyone.

279 If the snow is light and you can manage walking with good tread boots and warm clothing, push the snow in strips across your driveway or sidewalk. Use a lightweight shovel that has a broad base. Lifting a shovel full of heavy snow is too difficult. Hopefully, snow and ice will not prevent you from accomplishing light outdoor activities.

Out and About
(Tips 280–365)

Getting out of the house is the key to your recovery. The more you relate to others, the easier it will be to continue. It is a good idea to forget about stroke issues for a while. Put on your coat and get out of the house. You will be pleasantly surprised. Don't forget to bring your cell phone or smartphone.

Using a Smartphone, Cell Phone, or Telephone (Tips 280–292)

Post-stroke aphasia may delay our use of the phone when speaking. Technology can assist us to overcome some of these difficulties. (The irony of having a "smart" phone is not lost on me. I wish this technology would have been available when I was in school.)

280 **Install, or have someone help you install, an application (app) like Skype on your smartphone or computer** (if your computer has a camera—if not, you can purchase a camera add-on). This application allows you to see and hear your contact person, and they can see you too—in real time. For example, if you wish to contact your family or friends living elsewhere, but you are having difficulty talking, Skype is a great tool for them to see you and offer support.

281 **If you are able to verbally communicate when using a smartphone, use the speakerphone feature to amplify calls and improve flexibility.** When making or answering a call with a smartphone, there is a speaker icon (picture) located on the lower left portion of the phone. Lightly tap this icon and your call will be amplified for better hearing and communication. Also, the speakerphone feature allows you to put the phone down for improved coordination. Others may be able to hear the call as well so it is good to let the caller know he or she is on speakerphone.

282 **Keep frequently called numbers in your cell phone directory, or by your hard-wired phone.**

283 **If you primarily use a hard-wired phone, ask your telephone carrier to offer you free directory assistance because of your disability.** Most phone companies will provide this service after you complete an application process. Remembering several-digit numbers may be too difficult and telephone books have small print.

284 **Some hard-wired phone companies offer a telephone assistance plan for low-income disabled customers.** This may save you a little money on your monthly phone bill.

285 **Always have paper and pen or pencil ready.** Not everything is computerized these days.

286 **Those computerized answering systems are not user friendly.** When calling a company that has an automated answering system, tap or push "0" to get a representative as soon as possible or you will be barraged with complicated instructions. These systems can be complex for everyone. Too many instructions may cause stroke survivors stress and anxiety. It may be difficult to remember the purpose of the call when given various instructions.

287 **Keep phone conversations short and as uncomplicated as possible.**

288 **Ask your caller to send you the information via mail.** This way you can read and comprehend at your own pace or someone else can read it to you. You will avoid feeling pressured to agree to something over the phone that you may not remember later.

289 **Ask a family member to make a phone call for you.** Be sure to discuss the information you are requesting prior to the call.

290 **Practice phone calls with family members to rehearse your voice modulation and comprehension skills.**

291 **Make sure you understand how to operate your cell phone or smartphone.** Like a hard-wired phone, if you tap or press 911 but cannot speak, an ambulance will be summoned automatically if you just stay on the line.

292 **Keep your phone on a bedside table at night, within easy reach.**

Car Travel (Tips 293–296)

293 **Take your time when entering and exiting your car.** Hold the doorframe for support to assist you to a standing position, pivot toward the car seat, and sit down sideways. Then, swing one leg at a time into the car.

294 Buckle your car seat. Ask for assistance if necessary. Make sure you are buckled in before traveling in any motor vehicle. It's the law.

295 If you use a walker or a cane, make sure to take it with you when traveling.

296 A swivel seat cushion may be helpful for turning your hips and upper legs when getting into or out of a car. The North Coast Functional Solutions catalog offers swivel seat cushions like the one pictured.

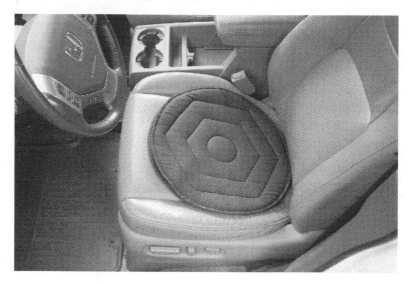

Airline Travel (Tips 297–306)

297 Keep your medication with you and in its original containers when traveling, especially when traveling by plane.

298 Pack light. Bring lightweight carry-on luggage that has wheels and a sturdy handle for pulling. A large canvas bag can hold your purse or other essential materials so you will be within the two-bag carry-on limit. Ask for lifting assistance when using the overhead compartments.

299 **If you're going on an extended vacation, check your luggage and carry just one bag or backpack with you**.

300 **Request a forward aisle seat when making a reservation**. When making reservations by phone, tell the representative that you have a disability and request a forward aisle seat. And whether you reserve by phone or complete this online, choose the seat that allows your affected side to face the window. This will help you to protect your affected side and aid in easier access to the toilet or in requesting assistance.

301 **Make mobility arrangements ahead of time** with the airline carrier for accommodations at your destination point and at any airport where you have to change planes. If you aren't using a wheelchair, a cart and driver can meet you and take you to your next destination. If you are in a wheelchair, an airline flight attendant or concierge service will take you to your next plane or destination within the airport, if you have made prior arrangements.

302 **If you are traveling in a wheelchair, your chair will stay with you until you transfer to the airline seat**. Then, it will be safely stored on the flight and ready for you when you land.

303 **All airline passengers with disabilities are allowed and encouraged to board the aircraft prior to standard passenger boarding**. This allows the flight attendant time to assist you.

304 **Use the toilet prior to boarding**, as it may be difficult for you to use the small cramped toilet facilities on the plane. But if needed, press your call button for a flight attendant to assist you.

305 If you need to use the airline toilet, tear off the toilet paper needed before sitting down so it will be more convenient. Make sure you hold onto the grab bars while situating yourself.

306 Moist towelettes or antibacterial hand wash help with easy clean up, as airline faucets flow only when you push the handle. Another alternative is to close the sink and fill a little water in the basin for easy hand washing.

Adaptive Recreation (Tips 307–340)

It's time to play. Find pleasure in activities you enjoyed doing before the stroke. You've worked hard, and will continue to work throughout your recovery process; now it's time to have fun. Almost all sports and recreational activities can be modified to support people with disabilities. Here are just a few:

Adaptive Gardening

307 Use adaptive equipment such as pulleys for hanging baskets and bird feeders.

308 Use roll out strips that contain flower seeds instead of planting seeds individually. Most local garden centers have these planted flower strips.

309 An alternative: place seeds on a strip of newspaper attached by a paste made from flour and water. Then plant the entire strip. It's biodegradable.

310 Modify the design by raising flowerbeds for easy reach.

311 Make garden paths wider. Easier for mobility.

312 Growing things vertically may be easier than horizontally. Use a trellis or lattice type fencing for flowers to grow up on.

313 Wrap foam pipe insulation around the hose nozzle and gardening tools for easier gripping. Ask for assistance if necessary. Purchase the foam pipe insulation that is already slit for easier application.

314 Use a small three-wheel pull cart (with pockets for tool storage hung on the outside) instead of a wheelbarrow.

315 Use foam packing balls or peanuts in the bottom of planters for proper drainage. They're lightweight, work great, and are easy to manipulate one handed.

316 Use a soaker hose or sprinkler for watering versus holding the hose.

317 Use a self-rewind hose. Avoid tripping over gardening equipment.

Adaptive Bowling

Most bowling centers have adaptable equipment available for bowlers.

318 An adaptable bowling frame is a lightweight aluminum frame that holds the bowling ball. The bowler places the ball on the frame, aims the frame at the pins, and rolls the ball down the frame's ramp. This style of bowling works great for stroke survivors.

319 **Gutter guards can be placed in bowling alley gutters to facilitate hitting the pins.** Try them when you first start bowling. Once you feel comfortable, move up to a more challenging game and bowl without gutter guards. Success comes in steps.

320 **Wear surgical booties over your street shoes.** Ask the bowling center management if this is allowed before you proceed. This will keep your ankle foot orthotics (AFO) in place during movement. Surgical booties can be obtained at any hospital supply store.

321 **If the previous tip is not possible, request two sizes of bowling shoes; one for your unaffected foot and a larger size to accommodate your AFO.**

322 **Seek assistance, if needed, when stepping up onto the bowling floor.**

Adaptive Golf

This is a game that has "handicap" and "stroke" as part of its terminology.

323 **Adaptive equipment and instruction is available.** Clubs, as well as nonswing clubs, balls, bionic gloves, and other adaptive equipment are available through your computer or smartphone worldwide web online information. Golf courses that assist adaptive golfers and offer instructors to help you get back in the swing again are available at many golf facilities.

324 **Practice swinging without a ball** in a large open space until you feel comfortable with the clubs again. You may discover your own adaptations.

325 **Practice at driving ranges and miniature golf courses to improve your swing and putting abilities**. Reducing expectations assists self-esteem as we work towards new techniques and goals.

326 **Use an adaptive golf cart**. If unavailable, use a regular golf cart but have your golfing partner drive. Go along for the ride.

327 **Use a modified swing for accuracy**. Your golf game may begin with a higher score, but play for technique at first.

Adaptive Fishing

328 **Some states offer free permanent fishing licenses for disabled individuals**. Check with your state fish and wildlife agency.

329 **Always wear a flotation device if fishing from a boat**. It's the law.

330 **Use an easier style fishing pole**. Check with your local sports shop.

331 **Fish from shore or a pier if you have any difficulty with balance or dizziness**.

332 **If you fish from a small boat**, get into the boat from a dock (pier) by sitting on the dock, placing your feet into the boat and sliding from the dock to the middle seat of the boat.

333 **Purchase a harness to hold your fishing pole** against your body in order to manipulate the reel with one hand.

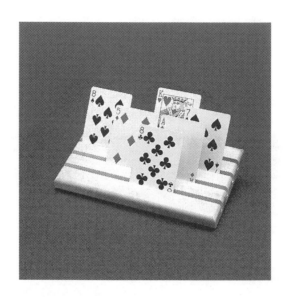

Adaptive Card Playing

334 **Use a large deck of cards.** They are easier to hold and see the suits and numbers.

335 **Play simple games at first and advance** to more difficult games as your memory and tactile skills improve.

336 **Play solitaire on a computer** to easily manipulate the cards as you relearn suits and numbers.

337 **Computer games, while easier to play, can also lead to isolation.** Use them sparingly. Socialization is a key factor in recreation and stroke recovery.

338 Use a finely sanded block of wood with a groove cut in the middle to hold your cards. (Use the block of wood described in Nail Care tip #156.)

339 You won't miss your turn at dealing if you have an automatic card shuffler. (They are available through adaptability catalogues, like North Coast Functional Solutions.)

340 To deal the cards manually, spread them on the table in front of you so that they are all in your visual field. Use your fingers to count out the cards and slide them to other players. Turn your head to get a good view of all the players if you have visual difficulties.

Driving After Stroke (Tips 341–354)

When will I be able to drive again? For many people independence hinges upon their ability to operate a motor vehicle. Transportation is a monumental task after stroke. Stroke survivors don't want to be a burden on others for this time-consuming job, especially if they were able to drive before having a stroke.

Why is it so difficult after a stroke? A simple answer is that stroke affects the brain. Driving is a serious task after a stroke, and the most dangerous one you may encounter during recovery.

341 Having a driver's license doesn't necessarily mean you are able to operate a vehicle after a stroke. A driver's license is used for identification purposes too.

342 You are responsible for using your license correctly. If you drive post-stroke without prior approval of your physician or attending an assessment program, you may be placing yourself and others at risk as well as jeopardizing the ability of your car insurance to cover damages should there be an accident.

343 Your neurologist or current physician will determine when and if it is practical and advisable for you to take on the responsibility of getting behind the wheel again.

344 If your physician agrees, he or she may refer you to a driving assessment program in your community.

345 What is a driving assessment program? A driving assessment program includes testing for comprehension, dexterity, visual field difficulties, thinking, memory, and judgment as well as other mandatory driving abilities. Part of this assessment includes a behind-the-wheel driving test. Your car may need adaptive equipment to compensate for stroke difficulties. An assessment program will offer suggestions. When you pass the assessment test, you will receive a certificate.

346 Where? Is there a cost? Check with your rehabilitation facility for a certified driving-assessment program near you. Prices can vary. Some programs offer a sliding fee for qualified recipients.

347 Take or send a copy of your driver's assessment certificate to your car insurance company. You may feel more comfortable about your achievement if it's on record.

348 The Department of Motor Vehicles has its own qualifications to drive: Among them are passing a vision test when your license is renewed and a requirement that a driver must be seizure free for 6 months before driving again.

349 Driving is multitasking! Your recovery is going so great that you are finally ready to do many things at the same time. But wait! There's more! The more you drive the better you get at it, just like when you were younger. Right? Not necessarily.

Plasticity is different than neuron growth in a normal adolescent's brain. Basically, a teenager may not have to contend with regrowth, but new growth.

Stroke recovery is a slow process. Much like the teen driver, your entire attention must be focused on driving. It may be frightening to steer, watch your speed, notice and react to other cars, pedestrians, and objects around you, while, at the same time, follow traffic rules and remember where you're going. Unlike the teenage driver, reaction times may be stilted and/ or half the vision of both eyes may be impaired necessitating turning our heads—if we remember to do so. Other medical conditions can add to the difficulties of multitasking.

350 **Pull over and rest when tired**. Many stroke survivors are on high alert when driving. It may be impossible to listen to music, a passenger, and focus on driving simultaneously. This extreme tension causes tiredness.

351 **Consider hiring a car service, or taking mass transportation or taxi service** if you live in an area with heavy traffic.

352 **Never use a cell phone while driving**. Cell phone use while driving is illegal in most states. Let's not tax the brain into doing more than humanly possible.

353 **A cell phone or smartphone can be handy if you have car trouble**. Make sure you are parked in a safe, well-lit area before using it.

354 **A smartphone can help you with directions**. Before driving, tap the front of the phone by the microphone icon. Speak into the phone, "driving directions." Speak your destination. Another way is by finding the app for Google maps. Type in the address of your destination. The smartphone will talk you through every turn. There is no need to hold the phone while using these apps either. Just swipe after you've reached your destination.

Restaurant Dining
(Tips 355–359)

355 **Opening containers are difficult one handed.** Small containers of butter, creamers, jelly, and sugar can be tricky. Ask for assistance from a server in a restaurant.

Place them within easy reach on your unaffected side so you can see them. Don't forget to leave a nice tip for this added service.

356 **You might request the food to be cut up in small pieces when you're ordering it.** Restaurants will provide this service for you and you will feel more independent.

357 **You may also want to order soft food to avoid any chance of choking.**

358 **If you have visual field difficulties,** hold the menu on your unaffected side so that you can see the entire fare.

359 **If you have visual field difficulties, turn your plate to notice food on your affected side.**

Invisible Disability
(Tips 360–365)

Some stroke survivors may indicate only slight spasticity or other viewable difficulties after stroke. To others, it may look as if nothing at all has happened. This can be a double-edged sword regarding disability issues. There are times when you may feel comfortable enough to discuss your disabilities with others and times when you do not feel that disclosing this information is advantageous to you. No one should take that right away from you.

360 **If you are aphasic or cannot communicate clearly**, there are cards available from the American Heart Association/ American Stroke Association that explain aphasia and you may distribute them as you see fit.

361 **You have two choices** when in the presence of people with closed minds. You can either avoid them or take on the responsibility to enlighten them about stroke. This may be a difficult task, so be prepared. You can start with, "I've had a stroke. Stroke is a brain attack. I would appreciate your tolerance and understanding. There are many hidden disabilities related to stroke. Do you know anyone who has had a stroke?" Let them respond. Chances are that they do.

362 **Make no apologies for a disability**, but do apologize if you have said something or done something that has offended someone. Sometimes stroke survivors lack a filter. We may have difficulty thinking before we speak. We may not even be aware that our comment was hurtful to others. We may change the topic of conversation rapidly because something just popped into our heads. Holding the focus of conversation may be difficult after stroke.

363 **Do not be apologetic about your right to use the law to assist you**. There may be times when you desire to keep your difficulties to yourself. Under the Americans with Disabilities Act of 1990 you are protected against discrimination in the workplace, afforded appropriate accommodations, and have civil rights to accommodations in public places, including transportation and telecommunications.

Pending your physician's approval and a small registration fee from The Department of Motor Vehicles (DMV), you may have a disability license plate on your car or display a disability placard when parking. This is your right. Many people before you have fought for this accessibility issue.

I have a disability placard for my car. Especially in the winter, I park the car in a disability space and use it. Many times I have encountered glares from others who disapprove of my parking because I may not look disabled to them. I don't know them and owe them no response. Countless trips to the emergency room have occurred because of falls happening post-stroke. If some accidents can be avoided by parking closer to an entrance or in a wider space so you can step out without slipping or have enough space to accommodate an adaptive device, so be it.

364 **If you and your physician agree to your returning to the workplace or pursuing other employment opportunities, you are under no obligation to disclose your disability to your employer**. You may, however, request special accommodations to help you perform the tasks expected of you. Whether you disclose or decide not to disclose, it is your decision. Remember, too, that as stroke survivors we may think we can do more than we are actually ready or able to accomplish. Be kind to yourself and gradually work up to your potential.

365 **Social Security Disability Insurance is managed on a case-by-case basis**. Some stroke survivors may be able to return to work; some may need to explore other positions; and some may not be able to return to the workforce.

Relaxation
(Tips 366–393)

There are powers in your mind that cannot be altered by medical intervention—a strong sense of self. Honor the dignity of your being. This may involve overcoming barriers we set ourselves by repeating the "I can't" mantra. In this chapter, addressing the control you own will be discussed.

Mindfulness, Meditation, and Guided Imagery (Tips 366–380)

"Mindfulness" is a simple invitation to live in the moment. This technique of relaxation embodies a sense of calmness by practicing silence, contemplation, and being attentive to our needs by allowing our bodies and minds to relax. It involves becoming consciously aware of our breathing, heartbeat, sensations, and measured movement.

366 **Mindfulness training is an alternative to numbing our feelings with medication.** However, check with your physician before tapering off any antidepressant medication. Learn relaxation techniques first, and then discuss taking fewer antidepressant medications with your doctor. There may be side effects of not taking the antidepressants as prescribed.

367 **Open your mind to new techniques**. They will prevent pushing your body and mind to exhaustion.

368 **Meditation and guided imagery will help you to continue working on adaptation skills and exercises at home**. Meditation and guided imagery are designed for anyone who wants to assist the body's natural tendencies to repair and heal. Both of these complement medical treatments. By using your mind to help you relax, you may feel stronger and improve more quickly.

369 **These techniques are targeted to help alleviate pain, reduce high blood pressure, boost the immune system, and relieve anxiety, stress, and depression.**

370 **There are many audio versions of guided imagery, aimed specifically for stroke survivors,** available through bookstores and online.

371 **Guided imagery is best performed at night,** just as you begin to sleep, when you are quiet and relaxed.

372 **Meditation can be done anytime and anywhere that is quiet and peaceful**.

373 **With all relaxation techniques, if your mind begins to wander, acknowledge the thought and gently sweep it away;** off stage, in the wings of your mind's theatre.

374 **You may feel unexpected emotions**. If this happens, allow the feelings to come up and move through you, seeing it as a necessary cleansing that is taking place. It won't hurt you to do this. Emotional healing is positive, not negative.

375 **Commit to this daily process,** engaging the power of your mind to help you heal and gently immerse yourself in this safe, inexpensive, and easy process.

376 **Relaxation exercises can replace negativity and conflict.** Let everything go and just be. Stroke survivors can get so emotionally and physically involved in the recovery process that we forget to allow our brains and thinking processes of the mind time to unravel and totally relax.

377 **Take a slow cleansing breath** by inhaling as fully as possible through your nostrils, engaging your abdomen with the breath. Then slowly, and with purpose, imagine sending the warm energy of your breath to any part of your body that is tense or tight. Release the discomfort with the exhale. Repeat this slow, deep breathing process. This is only the beginning of the process of deep relaxation.

378 **Meditation or guided imagery takes the power away from stroke as we begin to empower ourselves.** Relaxation techniques are designed to tap into the subconscious. Your subconscious will help you heal by giving you more inward strength, energy, and power as you learn to release and experience each moment by being present. With practice, you will become aware of each breath, as you quiet your mind to mentally picture your entire body— even your affected side.

379 **Stroke-specific guided imagery uses descriptive language to take you to a place of comfort and imagination that allows you to experience strength you might not know you possess.**

380 **Emotional feelings like resentments, harsh expectations, and unrealistic demands begin to dissolve with practice and time.** This allows stroke survivors to ease up on themselves and slow down. Without judgement, forgive yourself and others for disappointments of the past; let it all go.

Gentle Yoga/Chair Yoga
(Tips 381–386)

Yoga is widely practiced for health and relaxation. Gentle yoga is another form of mindfulness or meditation. In gentle yoga, modifications eliminate unnecessary strains on our bodies. Gentle yoga postures are low impact. However, some postures, or poses, can be more challenging than others. The positions are centered on your breathing as your body relaxes into each movement. Chair yoga, using the same principle, is yoga practiced while seated.

"Namaste" (pronounced na-ma-stay) means "I bow to the divine in you." There are many other interpretations as well. This word is used at the end of a yoga practice or after meditation. Seeing others through the definition of Namaste will help you to see the true divine spirit in everyone. Think of it as a blessing that honors the wholeness and equality in everyone. Stroke survivors thrive on honor and blessings.

381 **Take a gentle yoga, or chair yoga, class led by a certified yoga instructor.** She or he will teach you the art of easy postures that will help you feel comfortable. Although there are many yoga DVDs and computer streaming videos available, class instructors will help you adapt in ways that will not cause discomfort. In so doing, you may enjoy the practice. Also, some poses may not be appropriate or safe for you at the beginning. More importantly, by attending a gentle yoga class, you are getting out of the house and joining a group.

382 **There are many gentle yoga, or chair yoga, poses (positions) for you to try.** All you need is a yoga mat for gentle yoga, a chair for chair yoga, comfortable clothing, and a yoga instructor.

383 **If transportation is an issue for you, contact a transportation service in your area.** There are many available services such as bus, taxi, disability services, and paratransit services for the disabled and elderly that use adapted vehicles, and provide mobility services. You may want to connect with the social services department of your rehabilitation facility for other options. Another great place to look for transportation options, or yoga classes in your area, is through your local stroke support group.

384 Gentle or chair yoga classes may be provided by your local hospital, through their Wellness or Health and Fitness Center. This would be an excellent place to start. These facilities provide certified instructors and have therapists on staff to help you, if needed.

385 Gentle yoga, or chair yoga, may be offered through your neighborhood church or synagogue. Many places of worship offer community outreach for their members or the public. Sometimes there is a small fee to cover the cost of instruction, but others may offer this service free of charge.

386 Health insurance companies may cover most, if not all, of your monthly membership fee to join a qualified health or fitness center. Staying active and fit is the cornerstone of health insurance.

Music (Tips 387–389)

387 Music is profoundly useful. Some stroke survivors that have lost the ability to speak can relate a few words to the beat of music or are able to sing. Other benefits of music therapy are noted in movement and mobility improvements. Depression and anxiety are decreased in stroke survivors who listen to music on a regular basis. When listening to music, focus on the sound. Concentrate on the instruments' crescendos and tempo.

A note of information: Composer Johann Sebastian Bach and past vocal artists such as Cab Calloway, Luther Vandross, Mel Tormé, and Isaac Hayes had strokes. Today, soloists Brett

Michaels, Randy Travis, and singer/actress Della Reese are living well after stroke.

388 **Whatever type of music you enjoy may take your mind off of stroke.** If you are able to use a computer or smartphone, you can purchase your favorite tunes as downloads.

389 **If you play an instrument,** check with your local community college music department for a class that will provide for adaptation so you can play one handed. Private lessons are another option. I play right-handed piano.

Mirrors (Tips 390–393)

Visual spatial difficulties happen when a stroke affects the parietal lobe of the brain where our spatial mapping is located. This condition is also referred to as: "neglect." A stroke survivor may not be aware of objects on their affected side or, in some cases, realize there is a left side of the body. The difficulty lies in the brain's inability to process information correctly.

Mirrors are essential to your recovery process because they afford a practice of using your visual and spatial acuity. We won't recognize what we don't see. If we have left or right visual or peripheral field difficulties, a mirror is a safe place to learn to turn our heads in order to see both sides of the body. Have several sizes, including a full-length mirror, at your disposal.

390 **Mirrors help you to realize that you are indeed a whole person.** Mirrors help to control arm and leg movements too. Mirror boxes used in therapy stimulate the brain by reflecting an image of the unaffected side of the body. Thus, tricking the brain into thinking that both sides function.

391 **A mirror exercise**. Look into a large mirror. While keeping your head stationary, look to the left. What do you see? Look to the right. What is reflected in the mirror? Can you name the things you saw while looking straight ahead?

392 **Now, it's time for facial exercises**. Smile as broadly as you can. Pucker your lips. Stick your tongue out and move it slowly to the right and left. Close one eye then the other. Put your lips together as if you are blotting your lips. Open your mouth as far as possible and then close it. Blow to make your lips flutter. Move your tongue and pouch out one side of your mouth and then the other. Raise one eyebrow and then the other. Try to make individual vowel sounds. For stroke survivors with aphasia, practice simple words like "boat," "car," or colors, and opposite words like "stop" and "go" and try saying your name. All these facial exercises help orientate new brain neuron development and assist you in reclaiming your vital personality that shows through your face.

I practiced these techniques daily and, over time, it has assisted me indirectly with applying makeup, learning to smile again, learning to move my eyes and head to see missed objects, and perhaps most importantly, has improved my self-esteem.

393 **A full-length mirror can assist you in viewing your affected side for proper dressing and grooming as well**.

Brain Builders
(Tips 394–469)

Organization (Tips 394–401)

Organization assists our minds in healing. Disarray bombards our senses with overstimulation.

394 **Keep a journal** of your progress and add important information, like medications and doctor's phone numbers, to the entries too.

395 **Keep important information at hand.** An accordion file works well for keeping hospital information, therapy handouts, and information about stroke support groups. A different colored file can hold medical bills.

396 **Aphasic stroke survivors require a communication board, letter board or notebook, and pens at ready access.**

397 **A small digital voice recorder or tape recorder (old technology still works) will aid memory.** Organizing our thoughts is important too.

398 **Pack away items you do not frequently use**. Make room in your life (and brain) for current issues. Allow a family member to review the items before being stored so they can help you remember what is packed. A list of items may be helpful.

399 **Sticky notes can add to confusion**. Replace small adhesive sticky notes with a notebook and pen or a computer tablet placed in a specific central location where you can jot down necessary information.

400 **Keep appointments on a calendar**. The calendar should be in an obvious place you see every day. A calendar will help orient you to month, date, and year too.

401 **Try to avoid major changes in your life, at least for the first year post-stroke**. You've already had a major change. If you can avoid moving to a new location, changing legal paperwork like a will or signing legal documents, and so forth, do it. These add stress and another upheaval to stroke recovery.

Exercising (Tips 402–407)

As stated previously, the adage "move it or lose it" highly applies to stroke recovery. If neurons are not trained to travel new pathways within the brain, new connections will not be made and the stroke-affected side will get weaker and weaker as the unaffected side becomes stronger. Formal therapy is our beginning point, but we must take the techniques learned in rehabilitation home and continue to exercise our affected areas.

402 **Good posture is imperative**. Sit up straight and arch your back every once in a while. Drop your shoulders and stretch your neck so that your head is erect. Stroke-affected areas feel heavy resulting in the body slouching under the strain.

Good posture techniques decrease this tendency and remind the brain of the duality of our body.

403 **Move your feet when sitting**. Try to put both feet together on the floor when sitting. Then, move the unaffected foot out a few inches and try to have the affected foot follow. Now try placing the unaffected foot back, followed by the affected foot. This exercise won't work if your "adaptive technique" is to hook the affected foot with the other foot. Try sliding the affected foot by moving your knee and lower leg.

404 **This exercise helps alleviate foot drop** by building the muscles in the foot and training the brain to recognize both feet. When sitting, lift your toes up as far as possible while your heels remain on the floor. This little foot dance can be improvised too: one foot at a time, or both feet.

405 **Try climbing the wall**. Stand close to a wall. Your affected side should be near the wall. Spread your feet out for improved balance. If necessary, hold onto the back of a sturdy chair for balance. Place your affected hand, palm spread if possible, on the wall. Use your fingers to slowly climb your hand up the wall as far as possible. Have a family member place a small pencil mark on the highest point you can reach. Try to reach higher each day. Move very slowly at first, as this exercise can be difficult.

406 **Try this balance-training exercise.** While holding on to the back of a sturdy chair with one hand, look straight ahead and shift your weight from one leg to another. When you feel steady, lift one leg by bending your knee. Try to stand for 15 seconds without putting your foot down. Lower your leg and repeat on the other side of your body. Try this exercise without the chair when you feel ready to do so.

407 **If you like exercise videos**, there are many available for stroke survivors on the Internet as well as other formats. The

American Heart Association/American Stroke Association has exercise videos available for stroke survivors too. (The AHA/ASA is listed in the Resources of this book.)

Television Brain Power (Tips 408–412)

408 **Selective television viewing can be beneficial and regenerate brain power**. Quiz shows like *Jeopardy, Family Feud*, and others, as well as programming available on the Public Broadcasting System (PBS), like *Nova*, will not turn you into a couch potato.

409 **Quiz shows that have multiple choice answers (where you can see, read, and hear) are best for playing along**. An example is *Who Wants to be a Millionaire*.

410 *Jeopardy*, **in which you must phrase your answer in the form of a question, may be more difficult**. If you know the answer, try saying it without forming a syntactical question. Try not to think too hard but say the first thing that pops into your mind. If you're involved in the game, you may not be as self-conscious about any speech difficulties you may be experiencing.

411 **Be creative and invent your own television-viewing brainpower**. Here's one I discovered. Try to remember as many advertisements as you can between programs. Mute the television, close your eyes, and try to recall the products being sold in as many advertisements as possible.

412 **Who's on first?** is another memory retention made-up game. Try to remember the scheduling of your favorite show. What is the name of the show? What time does it come on? What day of the week? What is it about? Who's your favorite character? Who plays that character? This adds to your thinking, retention, and social skills.

Technology (Tips 413–423)

Smartphones are wonderful devices. This minicomputer not only performs well as a phone, but stores frequently called numbers, contact information and e-mail addresses, offers Internet access, allows for social media, text messages, e-mails, music, photograph capture and storage, and the list goes on. Another great feature of some smartphones is their capacity to perform voice messaging, access information, send e-mails, take notes, or give driving directions just by talking into them. This is advantageous for stroke survivors who need assistance with typing or writing.

The drawback is in their overuse. For example, some people gather at a table for a meal and never look up from their devices. People use them while driving, which is illegal, and many people have been killed or injured using a smartphone or cell phone in this manner. Even walking and texting isn't very smart.

People are in accidents every day because they are trying to multitask. Most stroke survivors instinctively know how difficult multitasking can be and avoid taking on such responsibility. Therefore, unless logical thinking is a bit askew, it can be noted that many stroke survivors have more common sense than many people who have not had a stroke.

413 **Do one thing to the best of your ability. Then, move on to the next task.** Isn't this the way things should be done for everyone? Learning to slow down can have its advantages.

414 **Computers make life easier**. There are software programs that help you with almost anything. For a small additional monthly fee through numerous service providers, you can "surf the web." Larger monitors (viewable screens) are available to assist visual problems.

415 When using Internet search engines on a smartphone or computer, make sure the sites you view (visit) are from professional and respectable authorities. The ending of a website .org (organization) or .edu (education), or gov. (government) will give insight to their legitimacy. There is so much information available on the World Wide Web that it may be confusing to find a reputable source.

416 Social networking can be a great place to meet others and to keep up with friends and relatives. Social networks allow stroke survivors throughout the world to connect, meet in support groups, and discuss topics important to their specific recovery. Perhaps you are having a particular problem that others are experiencing too. You're not alone.

417 Keep a journal of your recovery on your computer. When it is kept in a file on a computer, you can easily go back and read previous entries to see how far you have progressed. Also, using the keyboard in typing, reading the written word, and gathering your thoughts are all part of stroke recovery.

418 The bad news is that working at a computer is usually a solo activity. It is easy to get so engrossed in doing an activity that users forget there is a world about them to be explored.

419 Basic computer classes are available through community education classes, local business schools, or universities. Enjoying what your community has to offer is good toward stroke recovery too.

420 Don't be afraid to play with your computer. Open a software program and experiment with the wonderful opportunities and choices it offers. The best way to learn is by doing. Stroke survivors have a great capacity to learn new technology too.

421 **Voice recognition software** allows the computer to type the words you say and works with a microphone headset. It may take some time in training the software to recognize your voice and correctly spell the words you desire, but after you become familiar with the program, it could be a good tool for you.

422 **Financial management software is available too**. Online banking and your bank's bill-pay option is surely a time saver. After someone teaches you the bill-pay process, it will be much easier than writing checks, stuffing envelopes, finding stamps, and mailing. Online banking keeps records of your transactions, so it is easier to remember.

423 **Computers, tablets, and smartphones have the ability for games too**. Gaming is a popular source of entertainment for many stroke survivors, from virtual reality games to more simplified solitaire and everything in between. Many games help stroke survivors with dexterity, memory, vision, and comprehension, all while having fun.

Returning to Work (Tips 424–429)

You and your physician will determine when you are ready to return to the workplace.

424 **There are two alternatives available through Rehabilitation Services for returning to your job or after you have found other employment**. The first is called "transitional" and the second is "supportive" employment. Transitional services offer part-time employees the short-term assistance of a job coach contracted through your local Rehabilitation Services. Supportive employment measures include a Rehabilitation

Services job coach who will work with you for an extended time to ensure you understand required tasks, your work environment, and appropriate work ethics.

425 **If you are able to return to your workplace,** check with your employer to see if you can do your work from home and correspond via your home computer. This will not only save travel time and expense but conserve your energy too. If you decide this route is for you, make sure you stay active outside of the home as well.

426 **Other jobs may be available within your former employment.** Some jobs may not be as stressful. If your employment benefit package remains unaltered, it may be advantageous for you to take a salary cut while recovering.

427 **If you're unable to return to your job,** check with rehabilitation services offered in your area for retraining or educational opportunities.

428 **Another option is the National Stroke Association's Return to Work (RTW) Toolkit** available online at www.stroke.org/rtwtoolkit offering an employment-readiness assessment quiz.

429 **Stroke can be very complicated.** It may not be just one area that is affected, like thinking skills or memory, but involve the ability to speak, move, understand, and countless other brain functions. In many cases, Social Security Disability Insurance may be the only option. Then, our full-time job is to work on improvement.

Home Office (Tips 430–440)

430 **A home office might be a great way for you to complete volunteer work or paid jobs.** However, check with your neurologist first to find out what adaptive measures he or she recommends for your work routine. The drawback is the isolation associated with working at home.

431 **If you tire easily and your attention span is limited, a home office provides for short work periods and the opportunity for comfortable rest.**

If you decide to implement a home office, here are some tips:

432 **Designate a room on the main floor of your home.** Avoid treacherous stairs. Convenience is key.

433 **Hire someone to install a wide L-shaped desk with plenty of open work space.** Card tables are too unstable. Safety and convenience are the objectives in recovery. The L shape will encourage you to look in both directions. Install a wall mirror above the desk on your affected side. This will assist you in adapting to your visual field.

434 **Place a desktop or laptop computer in the corner of the desk area. Make sure computer peripherals, such as printers and scanners, are nearby.** Other useful items are a digital voice recorder for that sudden burst of enlightenment, a paper shredder, and a copy machine. Check each installation, so that it is convenient for your unaffected side.

435 **Other furnishing you may need** are a comfortable high back chair for support and window treatments like mini blinds or other easily accessible blinds that can be cleaned and operated with one hand.

436 **Organize office supplies on a Lazy Susan, and within close reach.** A revolving tray is easy to operate one handed.

437 **A phone with a built-in speaker.** Some hard-wired phones have large buttons to make the numbers more convenient.

Use a headset on your telephone, if you use the phone frequently. To facilitate concentration, have calls forwarded into voice mail or a messaging device.

438 **Use your computer to type frequently used telephone numbers in a large, bold font, print them, place the sheet of paper in a picture frame, and hang it directly above your desktop computer**. Better to be safe than sorry, if an electrical outage occurs. The numbers are much easier to see this way too.

439 **Keep material close to you to avoid unnecessary steps**. Use stackable bins on wheels to store frequently used objects. Open bookshelves are great for storing reference materials. Keep frequently used material within your visual field.

440 **Here are some ideas for home office use**: newsletter contributor, E-Bay seller, marketer and seller of your handmade items on the Internet, online student, and your expertise combined with a new implementation or your business plan, website, or blog.

Hobbies (Tips 441–446)

Being able to continue with your favorite hobby, or taking up a new one after a stroke, can keep you physically and mentally active. Depending on the impact of stroke, it is important to find an enjoyable hobby that builds self-esteem and brings satisfaction to your life.

Gardening is both a great hobby and an outdoor recreational activity. (See Chapter 6, tips 307–317.)

441 **Painting can be an alternate form of expression for stroke survivors**. An easy beginner water color kit, large-grip brush, and small easel with a clip to keep the paper in place is a great and inexpensive way to start.

442 **Photography can improve eye-hand coordination**.

443 **Ceramics affords the opportunity to manipulate clay on a wheel using your unaffected foot, use a kiln, and paint the final creation.**

444 **Keep an object stable by using adhesive suction cups, sticky mats, chip-clip holders, or picture-hanging strips while you work with one hand**. This is handy for painting a bird house or doing anything that requires a stationary surface.

445 **Woodworking hobbies can be enjoyed too**. If you tinkered in a woodshop before the stroke, you may be able to return to your hobby with assistance and some adaptability safety efforts.

446 **Return to what you liked doing**. If you sew, knit, or make flower arrangements, you can do it post-stroke too.

I have a blue knit hat in my closet. It is the ugliest hat you'll ever see, but I love my hat. A year after the strokes I had, a friend gave me circular knitting needles, a pattern for a hat, and a skein of yarn and, without a word, left me to figure it out for myself. I had very little use of my left arm and fingers. How did she expect me to do it? I knit frustration, anger, tears, and, finally, adaptability into that hat. It took a long time, but I finished it. The hat has numerous dropped stitches resulting in holes, but this hat catapulted me into knitting again. Within the last 20 years, I have knit blankets, scarves, sweaters, numerous nicely knitted hats, mittens, novelty items, and fingerless gloves, and I've even made up my own patterns. But that ugly blue hat will always be my personal favorite. I have found that knitting is great for finger dexterity as well as fine motor development. My friend, a nurse, knew it before I did.

Talents (Tips 447–449)

447 **Adult coloring books relieve stress by offering a calming activity**. This activity requires small muscle movement and eye and hand coordination.

448 **Eye and hand coordination can be improved by using your ability to try new skills**. Some people enjoy putting together jigsaw puzzles; others enjoy completing crossword puzzles or word searches.

449 **Writing short stories takes creativity and computer-typing ability**. One hand can be used for the keyboard and the originality comes from you. It affords continuity in thinking skills.

Miscellaneous (Tips 450–458)

You've been invited to a party, where presents are expected.

450 **Make it easier**. Roll the gift in tissue paper, plop it in a bag, and place another piece of tissue in the bag so that the ends stick out.

451 **Another way to get a gift wrapped** is to order it online and have the gift sent to the recipient, gift wrapped, and with a card if desired.

Opening Compact Disc (CD) or Digital Versatile Disc (DVD) Packaging.

452 **Some adaptive devices can be used in various ways.** Place the CD/DVD in your kitchen cutting board vise grip. Use a sharp knife to cut the cellophane wrapping across one end and peel it off the rest of the CD/DVD. Placing it back in the vise, taped edge up, pry a knife tip under the tape to pull it off. Take the CD/DVD out of the vise and lay it flat with the opening to your unaffected side. Flip it open with the fingers of your unaffected hand.

453 **Another way, and my all-time favorite, is to have the store open the CD/DVD for you at the time of purchase.** Don't feel obligated to explain your disability; just ask them to open it for you. CD/DVD cases are difficult for everyone to open.

Clipping Coupons

454 **If you want to clip coupons out of the newspaper or weekly flyer for shopping, use a table or a wide, empty counter top for a surface.** Place a paperweight on the open newspaper to hold it in place. With the scissors slightly open, use the tip of the scissors as forceps to pick up the outer edge of the coupon. Don't worry if you don't do it perfectly the first time. This takes practice. The coupon will be accepted even if you cut a little wider than the dotted line indicated.

456 **Consider getting an app that allows you to scan coupons onto your smartphone.** First, check the Internet for your area stores' participation.

Tearing Paper Off a Roll.

457 **Take the amount you need and then, with the index finger and thumb of your unaffected hand, break the first few perforations of the paper.** Move the back of your hand up against the dispenser and proceed to break the remaining paper off the roll by using the same process, your thumb and index finger.

458 You want to write a note with your stroke-affected hand. Part of the difficulty may be in holding the pen or pencil and moving the hand.

Try using the Writing-Bird from North Coast Functional Solutions. By gently pressing on this lightweight device, the pen or pencil tip will glide along nicely.

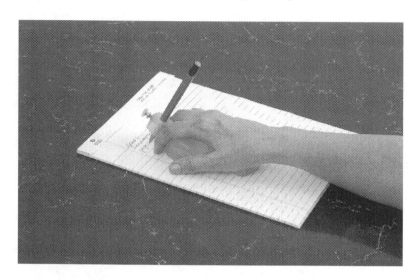

Pet Care (Tips 459–462)

Pet ownership is a big responsibility. Animals need daily care too. They need food, fresh water, exercise, frequent veterinarian checkups and immunizations, grooming, a city license if required, and lots of love.

If you have a pet that has been with you before you had a stroke, the animal may be a great comfort to you when you return from the hospital. However, there are some issues of pet ownership that you should be aware of after a stroke.

459 Be extremely careful that your pet does not trip you, or that you don't step on it. If you have a small dog or a cat, be aware that your pet may come up to you on your stroke-affected side and you may not be able to see it.

460 **Make sure you know where your small pet is before you use a walker or cane.** Your new equipment may appear to be a plaything to your animal.

461 **Your medical risk must be carefully weighed against the risk of getting a pet after stroke.** Will you be able to provide proper care for the animal? Will the pet interfere with your mobility? Will you be able to pet-proof your home? Does your apartment management accept pets? Who will care for the pet if you are away? Talk with a veterinarian about the care and feeding of a particular animal before you bring the new pet home.

462 **You are making, or have made, a major commitment to an animal and the responsibility for care is up to you.**

Games (Tips 463–469)

463 **Fast Naming**: This game builds language skills. Name as many things as you can in 1 minute. For example, name as many animals as you can in 1 minute. Name as many fruits as you can in 1 minute. Name as many things that are red in 1 minute. In 1 minute, name as many things that you can think of that are round. Use your own imagination or play the game with a few friends and time yourself.

464 **20 Questions**: Memory and critical thinking skills game. Someone writes down the name of an animal, person, or object. They state the category, whether it is an animal, person, or object. Then, individuals in the group ask 20 yes or no questions to determine the specific answer.

465 **Seven Words**: Verbal and creativity challenge. Use only seven words to tell a story.

466 **Get the Picture**: A visual memory skill. Study a picture in a newspaper, magazine, book, or online for a minute. Hide the picture or turn away from the picture and write down or tell the partner playing with you all the items you can remember from the picture. Your partner can give you cues if you need help, like "what is the object by the (name something in the picture)?"

467 **Board Games** provide companionship and aid comprehension—*Scrabble, Pictionary, Operation, Clue, Jenga,* checkers, and chess are just a few examples.

468 **Individual-Player Games** foster thinking and memory skills—try solitaire, crossword puzzles, word searches, and *Sudoku.*

These are just a few of the many games and activities you can do at home to have fun and foster plasticity within your brain. You don't always have to work at recovery. You can enjoy yourself and your family and friends while reaping the benefits of building brain power.

469 **Coins can work your body and mind**. Coins can be used to develop small muscle coordination as well. Try picking them up from a flat surface and placing them into a container by using your stroke-affected fingers and hand. Count the coins as you proceed.

Sexual Relationships (Tips 470–490)

Love begins with a touch, a look, a hug, a smile, a thought, and a need for intimacy. Every person requires some form of intimacy. Relationships begin in the heart.

Women may feel that they are not as appealing after stroke as they were before. Men may experience erectile dysfunction. Furthermore, some medications may have an effect on your libido.

470 **You are the same person as before the stroke,** even if you may be experiencing slight personality differences post-stroke.

471 **Reevaluate your marriage/partnership commitment**. What specific adjectives describe your marriage/partnership? Life partner, sharing, love, parenting, pledge, vow, promise, sexuality, faithfulness, and unity are all words that may be used to describe your devotion to each other. Continue to enhance your unity.

472 **An open discussion with your physician may alleviate your, and your partner's, concerns about resuming sexual intercourse.**

473 **Stroke may cause self-image difficulties**. Help your lover understand that you still love him or her. If your partner is experiencing emotional problems toward resuming sexual relations with you because of the stroke, consult a professional counselor.

Intimacy (Tips 474–485)

474 If the desire for sexual intercourse is intact, and not muted by your medications, verbalize your desire to your partner or, if you're more comfortable, try body language like touching, smiling, and eye-contact.

475 Emotions are expressed in many different ways, like kissing and cuddling.

476 Labels can destroy intimacy. Caregiver and stroke survivor may now equal husband and wife or lovers.

477 Sexuality begins in the brain. How you use what you have can make for a very satisfying sexual experience.

478 Relax. You and your partner will enjoy the experience more if both participants are less stressed.

479 Many people who have had a stroke go on to lead a very satisfactory sex life.

480 Have fun and enjoy yourself and your partner.

481 Share your feelings as well as your joys. Everyone has them.

482 A sex therapist may be helpful in explaining how you and your partner can satisfy each other's needs.

483 Consult your physician about medication for erectile dysfunction.

484 Try various forms of sexual stimulation for arousal such as extended foreplay or oral sex.

485 Practice safe sex. Use a latex condom to avoid sexually transmitted diseases (STDs) and autoimmune deficiency (HIV/AIDS). Protect yourself and your loved one.

Positioning (Tips 486–487)

486 Communicate to your partner what position is the most appropriate for relaxation, touch, and movement.

487 Lay on your unaffected side or back for better control and balance.

Touch and Sight (Tips 488–490)

488 Consider keeping the lights on. After a stroke, your loved one may not be aware of the stroke-affected side if it can't be seen. Movement will be easier with the light on.

489 Communicate to your partner exactly what part of your body has been affected by the stroke and request manipulation of the unaffected side.

490 Use hand movements and facial expressions to indicate pleasurable touch if you are having difficulty communicating because of the stroke.

Family Care
(Tips 491–512)

Family Members and Family Relationships (Tips 491–498)

Stroke affects family relationships too. Psychologists, neurologists, stroke medical and rehabilitation team members all agree that stroke profoundly impacts family dynamics. Suddenly, you become responsible for helping your loved one during stroke recovery while simultaneously carrying on with normal, routine activities and chores. If you are employed, dreams of early retirement may have vanished. While your mate is working at improving, you may be faced with handling family finances, shopping, watching children (if they're still at home), cooking, cleaning, washing and putting away laundry, and keeping on top of home maintenance.

This stressful situation is further complicated by your concern for your loved one's health and welfare, and your stamina regarding the long, healing process required for stroke recovery. You may hear remarks like, "It will take time to heal" or "In time, your loved one may improve" or your stroke survivor/loved one might say, "Give me time to figure this out on my own!" In your world, time may be in very short supply.

Your family dynamics and marriage have changed. Some changes came over the course of time, others directly from the stroke. No one understands how much stroke has affected your life as well as you and your partner. All marriages take work to stay strong. Communicate effectively. Ease back on taking everything on as your personal responsibility. Give as much responsibility, power, and freedom to your stroke survivor/partner as is safely possible. He or she may surprise you.

491 **Join a stroke caregiver support group through your local hospital or rehabilitation facility.** This will provide you with the opportunity to speak with others who are going through similar circumstances.

492 **Plan time for yourself.** An evening out with friends or even a weekend away relieves stress enormously.

493 **Exercise daily.** Walk around the block or join a gym or exercise facility.

494 **Make time for your hobbies and interests, as they remain vitally important.**

495 **Ask friends, neighbors, relatives, coworkers, or church members to visit and assist you once in a while.** Company will help both of you feel less isolated and alone.

496 **Empathy is good, but sympathy and pity don't help.** Your partner relies on your understanding and encouragement. Empathy is the ability to step into another person's shoes and feel his or her particular situation. John Steinbeck wrote, "It means very little to know that a million Chinese are starving unless you know one Chinese who is starving." That's empathy.

Sympathy is a feeling of caring and concern for someone accompanied by a wish to see them better off or happier. "I wish you would get better" or "I hope things improve soon." A sympathetic person is sincere but detached. This emotion makes the stroke survivor feel alone.

Pity is neither sympathy nor empathy but an emotion explained by such words as, "My poor spouse had a stroke." Pity has a negative undertone and can express feelings of condescension. Pity indicates feeling sorry or bad for someone. Pity should be avoided at all costs.

497 **Attend doctor visits with your stroke survivor**. Bring written questions along that apply to you too. Caring for someone who has had a stroke is an awesome responsibility and you will need help through this journey.

498 **Family members may go through denial too**. You may hear and comprehend the physician's words regarding your loved one's diagnosis but may try to remain positive. You and other family members see your loved one progressing. It is natural to feel that when your loved one is sent home from the hospital, he or she is, at least emotionally, the same as before the stroke. It is important to have a family discussion with the psychologist member of your stroke team before hospital discharge regarding cognitive problems the stroke survivor may still be experiencing.

Positive Support (Tips 499–501)

499 **Assist in giving responsibility back to your partner**. First, this technique takes the burden of responsibility from you. Second, it provides independence for your partner and spouse. Finally, it is a positive way to heal. By empowering your partner—who has survived stroke—with the task of meal planning or cooking (even if that means ordering out) or laundry or cleaning and so forth at least 1 day a week, you are involving him or her in family activities again.

500 **You are not responsible for your partner's feelings.** Stroke happened to both partners and their family.

501 **Use parroting techniques to assist communication.** "I hear you saying ..." or "It hurt me when you said ..." By repeating the words your partner communicates to you, language and the way words are spoken can aid communication.

Children of Stroke Survivors (Tips 502–512)

Here, we will address the reaction of young children to a parent or grandparent who has had a stroke. Children depend on adults. So much attention centers on the stroke survivor and other adults in the family unit that children are frequently forgotten as being a part of the healing process.

502 **Children might regress to bedwetting, daytime diapers, baby talk, whining, or other negative behavior after someone in their family unit has a stroke.** This is a normal reaction to a traumatic event in their young lives. Preschoolers keenly sense stressful situations, even if they don't understand the problem. Children need to feel secure.

503 **Spend time with your child on a one-to-one basis.**

504 **Crouch down to your child's level and address the child face-to-face when discussing important matters.** Little ones want to be included in everything.

505 **Explain what happened in terms your child can understand.** "Something isn't working well in [place familiar name of stroke survivor here] brain right now and that is why [she/he] has trouble working [his/her] arm and leg. [He/she] is working on getting better."

506 Give your child simple tasks, like folding washcloths or matching socks, so that he or she feels helpful too.

507 Make a simple chart for your child, and place stickers on it for daily positive behavior and accomplished tasks. When a child earns a small number of stickers, he or she wins a new book, for example. Avoid giving food, candy, or expensive toys as a reward.

508 Have your child assist the stroke survivor in your family, as much as is safe. This can include looking at books together, retrieving items, and so forth. Be creative and make it fun.

509 Children are adaptable too. Perhaps your child can show you or the stroke survivor a new approach to performing a task.

510 Answer children's questions honestly. If you don't know the answer, tell them that you don't know.

511 Children need hope. Children need to know that you will be there for them. Let your child know that you and your family are working together every day toward getting better.

512 Children can and do have strokes too. Children who have had strokes are miraculous in their adaptability.

Motherhood and Surviving a Stroke

There are women who have had a stroke during labor or delivery too. The infant needs immediate attention but mom is dealing with the aftermath of stroke. Many of these courageous women go on to fight stroke and embrace motherhood. Some women have recovered enough after stroke to become pregnant a second time and deliver a second healthy infant. Both categories of women deserve a medal of honor in the Stroke Recovery Hall of Fame. Think of all their responsibilities and accomplishments. Could you, one-handed, change a diaper on a squirming infant? Could you chase a toddler? Could you pick a baby up and hold the little one securely? These women could teach us a lot about stroke recovery. By keeping their eyes set on a selfless goal, they empower themselves.

Stroke Prevention (Tips 513–523)

Tips for Stroke Prevention (Tips 513–523)

Knowing your risk factors for stroke can significantly lessen your chance of another stroke. There are risk factors we cannot change like our age, sex, ethnic group, family history of heart disease (coronary or vascular), and stroke. People who have sickle cell anemia are also at a higher risk of stroke.

Here are some tips about risks of stroke that we have the power to change, now and in the future.

513 **High blood pressure** should be checked regularly, and see your physician for medical treatment.

514 **Diabetes mellitus** requires medical intervention, a modified diet, and insulin.

515 **Heart disease or atrial fibrillation** can be controlled by medication or surgery, and frequent medical check-ups.

516 High low-density lipoprotein (LDL; bad cholesterol) or low levels of high-density lipoprotein (HDL; good cholesterol) can be partially regulated by medications, diet, and exercise.

517 **Obesity** can be controlled by eating healthily and getting 30 minutes of cardiovascular exercise every day. This may include walking or any adaptable exercise routine that increases the heart rate.

518 **Smoking** is treatable by quitting. But it's easier said than done, as tobacco affects the receptors in the brain that crave this habit. Tobacco use doesn't relieve stress. Instead, it places the user into a frenzy because the brain receptors are so active. In fact, tobacco use increases stress, causes lung cancer and other pulmonary diseases, and the residual chemicals are carried through the bloodstream to the brain. There are ways to quit using. Attend counseling or consult clinics or hospitals in your area that offer free services for quitting tobacco use. Over-the-counter (OTC) nicotine replacement therapies such as gum or lozenges may also help. Talk with your doctor about nicotine patches. Stress reduction through meditation, yoga, an exercise routine, or fitness program will offer relief from tobacco cravings.

519 **Alcohol abuse** can be alleviated by treatment.

520 **Illegal drug use** is treatable through treatment and quitting. But it is the same as trying to quit tobacco because the brain receptors are being sabotaged by cravings. Nevertheless, treatment is the only solution to a long and happy life.

521 **Birth control pills** carry a stroke risk for women. Check with your physician.

522 **Hormone replacement therapies (HRTs)** carry a stroke risk too. Check with your physician about your particular risks.

522 **Severe, persistent, deep hiccups** are being explored as a new risk factor too. Researchers are trying to discover the correlation and cause, but it is enough to know that these types of prolonged hiccups could carry a risk factor for stroke.

523 **Transient ischemic attacks (TIAs) or mini-strokes** are the forerunner or warning signs of stroke. Recognize the warning signs and call immediately for medical assistance if they occur. TIAs can be treated and can reduce your risk of having a major stroke. Sometimes, the cost of an aspirin a day, or a few cents, can alleviate a lifetime of stroke recovery and a myriad of financial difficulties. However, do not take aspirin unless your physician has approved it for you, as it may cause side effects when mixed with other medications you are taking.

Prevention of another stroke is an essential part of stroke recovery. Stroke is not a disease, although it can be caused by cardiovascular (heart and blood vessel) disease.

Stroke is a time-loss-equals-brain-loss condition. Worldwide public education regarding stroke symptoms and what to do when they occur is vital. The National Stroke Association's (NSA) "Act F-A-S-T" campaign exemplifies stroke symptoms by stating:

Face drooping

Arm uncontrolled

Speech slurred or slow

Time is brain. Call 911 for emergency assistance.

Medical Aspect of Stroke

Stroke Centers

Primary stroke centers are hospitals that have been certified by the Department of Health or The Joint Commission as centers that comply with the latest hospital guidelines for stroke treatment.

In 2000, a group of stroke experts from the Brain Attack Coalition (BAC) proposed the creation of two types of stroke centers that would give "ultra-rapid" stroke care: primary and comprehensive. A comprehensive stroke center has specific abilities to receive and treat the most complex stroke cases. The majority of these highly regulated hospital designations are primary stroke centers. However, not every hospital in the nation is designated a primary or comprehensive stroke center. Sometimes, these hospitals will teleconference with other area or regional hospitals regarding a specific case and, possibly, transport the patient to the closest stroke center.

You have met your stroke care team at either a primary or comprehensive stroke center or at a rehabilitation hospital: physicians, neurologists, physiatrists (PM&R—Physical Medicine and Rehabilitation—physicians), psychologists, therapists, and nurses. Now you have been released to the care of one physician who will continue to help you as you continue to recover at home.

There are more stroke centers and comprehensive stroke centers available at hospitals than ever before. But if we do not recognize or do not continue to educate others about stroke symptoms and about receiving immediate medical help, the large gap between public education and the person experiencing stroke symptoms getting quick treatment will persist.

Stroke Research

The National Institute of Neurological Disorders and Stroke (NINDS) supports research on ways to enhance, repair, and regenerate the central nervous system. Scientists funded by NINDS are studying how the brain responds to experience or adapts to injury by reorganizing its functions (plasticity)—using noninvasive imaging technologies to map patterns of biological activity inside the brain, among other scientific studies.

Other NINDS-sponsored scientists are looking at brain reorganization after stroke and determining whether specific rehabilitative techniques can stimulate brain plasticity, thereby improving motor function and decreasing disability.

One advancement that is gaining promise is vagus nerve stimulation (VNS). This procedure is still in clinical trials for stroke patients, both in the United States and in Europe, at the publication of this book. VNS implants a device into one of the two vagus nerves in the chest. Small stimulations are sent to the brainstem, either in the form of tiny electrical spurts or medication or both. It is thought to help curb severe depression, lessen spasticity (muscle contractions), and accelerate neuroplasticity (the capacity for continuous alteration of the neural pathways and synapses of the brain and nervous system).

Researchers are experimenting with implantation of stem cells to see if these cells may help in stroke recovery. Scientists in the United States have discovered that bone marrow stem cells, even given directly into the arteries in order to cross the blood–brain barrier, do not transform into neurons or brain tissue. They did, however, discover a way to infuse stem cells safely. That is a milestone that occurred over the past few years. Also, they suspect that the earlier this procedure is performed, the better the results may become. More research is needed.

Thanks to advancing medical technology, robotics and wireless systems are implemented to aid our recovery. Telecommunication is being used in the field by emergency medical technicians (EMTs) who may suspect stroke and immediately notify a neurologist. These advances help stroke rehabilitation, as expedient diagnosing translates into shorter recovery periods and less money and heartache spent on long-term rehabilitation.

We rely on educational efforts that teach public awareness about the urgency and warning signs of stroke. We support research to develop medicines and medical technology for faster and appropriate treatment. The future of stroke depends on our global effort.

Frequently Asked Questions

Seven Questions From Stroke Survivors

1. I miss who I used to be. Why am I so different?

Stroke can, in many cases, affect our thinking processes, our memories, our sense of personhood, and our movement. We may still look the same to others, but have undergone dramatic changes. We mourn for the person we were before stroke. We miss the fact that our bodies do not respond as before, in a smooth and unthinking way. We miss the person we used to be, doing the things we took for granted before having a stroke. Ultimately, our emotions boil down to Elisabeth Kübler Ross's Five Stages of Grief:

1. Denial: "I didn't have a stroke. This cannot be happening to me!"

2. Anger: "Why did I have a stroke? It's not my fault. Who can I blame for this life-long disability?"

3. Bargaining: "Just let me live to see a grandchild or another special holiday. I'll do anything just to exist."

4. Depression: "I can't do anything. I can't fight this. I'm too sad to care about life."

5. Acceptance: "I'm at peace with who I am. I'm able to see that I am improving. I'm at peace with the future."

These stages happen over time, and we will slip back and forth between them. We may stay in one stage longer than another. Eventually, we realize that time changes everyone. Your children are not the same people they used to be: they are growing or grown. You are growing too: maturing emotionally and aging physically. Time does help us grow.

2. When will I get better?

We go to the hospital for stroke care, and expect the medical community to restore our health. In many cases, this works, as more people survive stroke today than in the past. However, we must reconcile the fact that during a stroke part of the brain dies.

Your physician knows your medical history and is the best person to offer advice. All too often the answer to the question, "When will I get better?" is vague. It may be something like, "It depends on your age, your related medical conditions, your stamina, the part of the brain that has been affected by stroke."

There is a deeper, more scientific answer. The brain is an organ containing 86 billion neurons and trillions of connective synapses. The brain contains "zettabytes" of information, more than all the computers in the world combined. If you think of the brain as the body's electrical system, then stroke causes a short in the electrical circuit. Messages to our arm, leg, speech center, vision, swallowing muscles, comprehension and memory areas, may get disconnected. And sometimes this disconnection causes seizures.

It is not what the brain is but what the brain does that is vitally important to our recovery process. The stroke-affected areas of the brain—those areas damaged by lack of oxygenated blood caused by a blood clot or cholesterol (in the case of an ischemic stroke) or those areas affected by pressure from a brain bleed (from a hemorrhagic stroke)—don't function.

Unless you received tissue plasminogen activator (tPA) within a 3- to 4-hour time limit of the onset of stroke symptoms or received the groundbreaking surgery to remove the clot in the cases of an ischemic stroke or had immediate surgery to stop the bleeding in the case of hemorrhagic stroke, the stroke-affected areas of the brain die. That's the bad news. The good news is that you can improve a little more each day by helping the neurotransmitters in your brain make new connections. You will dramatically improve from where you are today if you continue to work at recovery.

You are extremely fortunate. You are home. The areas of the brain that were affected by the stroke can be, to a large extent, rerouted to other areas through a process called "plasticity." The flexibility of the brain is constantly changing. Your sense of hearing, vision, touch, taste, and even smell along with your ability to move an affected body part, feelings of discomfort, and the ability to speak and comprehend will cross reference with other patterns and decode messages. Sometimes, these messages will get scrambled and result in central nerve pain or central nerve syndrome (CNP or CNS), sometimes referred to as "thalamic pain" if the thalamic gland is affected or if the main message center or clearinghouse of the brain is affected. But you will improve. Perhaps this book will help you on your journey.

3. Where did my friends go?

Your friends have lives too. They are continuing to care for their loved ones just like you are. Be kind. Your friends may not understand your recovery process. If you desire their company, invite them to your home. Plan a simple coffee time by sending out written invitations to your close friends stating a specific afternoon date and time. Tell them you miss their company and friendship.

It takes a friend to be a friend. Life is full of new friends and old friends, as well as acquaintances and coworkers. Isolation leads to depression. Depression slows our recovery, among other things. Join a book club, a hobby club, a knitting group, a senior center, a health and fitness center, a support group, a singles group—anything you feel comfortable being a part of in order to meet new people and have fun.

4. My spouse and family don't understand me. Why can't they understand what I'm going through? (See Chapter 10, "Family Care," tips 491–498.)

Your family has experienced stroke too, but in a different way. They have taken on the responsibilities that you once had in addition to their own. It is extremely difficult to lose family placement. If you're a wife and mother, you want to continue in that role and not be relegated to the role of a child. If you are a husband and father, you likely want to be the protector and provide for your family. Whatever role you had, whether it was outside employment, childcare, household duties, volunteer groups you belonged to, or other duties, you want to continue playing this part. Your family wants you to continue in your very important role too. They're grieving, and yes, probably shocked, by this sudden change.

And most likely your spouse and family don't understand what you are going through as you work toward recovery, because this is your journey. Still, they need you; you need them. This is the core of family relationships. Being able to encompass the entire family structure may be difficult for you, and you'll sometimes feel depressed. Open these topics of conversation with your loved ones. Listen closely. Talk to them without self-pity, and reassure them that you are taking positive steps to improve but it will take time and work to do so. Tell them you love them.

You have improved since hospitalization and will continue to recover. But this will not be a race; instead, it will be a slow progression. When you need assurance of your family role, ask them. Gently and quietly, take a little responsibility for your role in the family. For example, do the laundry, cook a meal, or vacuum. It will keep depression at bay, make you stronger, and add to your self-esteem.

5. When I get a cold or a virus I feel as if I'm regressing in stroke recovery. Why do I feel so tremendously tired, as if I'm having another stroke?

Your body is fighting a virus or infection. All your energy now fights the virus/infection. You will regress slightly, but after the virus/infection clears, you'll bounce back to where you were before getting sick. Remember to consult your physician regarding medications for fighting a severe cold, virus, or infection, and to determine the exact cause of your illness.

A virus may send you to bed for a period of time, so don't forget to move around, get up, and breathe deeply to prevent pneumonia. Drink lots of fluids and eat what you can. Chicken soup or broth is best.

6. I had a stroke in my arm and leg; it didn't affect my ability to think. What can I do to improve?

Stroke occurs only in the brain, but this can impact your arm, leg, face, speech, comprehension, and so on. The stroke may have cut off communication to your extremities, so they don't work like before. It is very difficult to realize that there is nothing wrong with your stroke-affected arm or leg. The only reason your arm, leg, shoulder, or entire side of the body isn't functioning properly, is because your brain isn't communicating effectively with that particular area. These affected brain areas are gone, and will not return. However, plasticity (a good thing, as you probably know by now!) within the brain will occur if you help your affected side to move. This process minimizes pain and encourages movement if begun early and continued every day. If you are unable to work with your affected side, through hospital therapy and at home, soon spasticity will make it difficult, if not impossible, to unfreeze the limbs because of muscle and tendon contractions. Read, research, join stroke support groups, get therapy, but above all keep moving your stroke-affected body parts.

7. You don't look like you've had such a bad stroke. (See the "Invisible Disability" section in Chapter 6, tips 360–365.)

Appearances can be deceiving. Sometimes I take this comment as a compliment to my long hard-fought recovery process. On the other hand, people who say this don't have the wisdom that neurologists do. Any stroke is bad because brain cells die. For example, there are roughly 22 billion neurons in the forebrain, which is where many strokes occur. Nearly 2 million neurons die each second a stroke remains untreated.

These types of judgments also stem from preconceived notions of what "stroke" is supposed to look like. Because I am able to talk, walk, think, and write better than I was able to when I first had the stroke does not mean I am completely healed. I am an example of medical breakthroughs and good therapy. I am an example of gut-wrenching survival and hard work.

Epilogue

Feeding messages into the brain, trying new tasks, and rebuilding the brain by using many of the techniques included in this book mean the brain will eventually figure out a way to grow new neuron receptors around the damaged areas. This will not happen quickly, but you will slowly see results. New brain cells regenerate daily and it is imperative to continue mental and physical exercises consistently, along with periods of rest, in order to train the brain to make those new connections. Time equals brain healing too. Use time to your advantage.

Our long-term brain health is ultimately our responsibility. As stroke survivors we are home from a long and frightening journey. Our recovery story is far from over. We are learning new ways of doing things. We exercise our mind, spirit, and body daily. We eat healthy to keep our body and mind strong. We rest when we are weary—which is often. We find enjoyment in social skills, hobbies, relaxation, and family relationships. We go back and forth between encouragement and depression. We work, full time, at recovery. It is a difficult job. You are trying to recover as much as possible after stroke. Keep trying. When the struggle seems overwhelming, relax, breathe deeply, and notice the little things in life.

Writing this book has brought me back to a very uncomfortable place in my life. I wasn't sure I wanted to return; to try to realize what it was like when I first came home from stroke rehabilitation. If I didn't, the writing would read very didactically—preachy and scientific—educational certainly, but not real. I have always been a little suspect of people telling me what to do if they have never experienced what I was going through at the time. Talking about stroke issues is one thing; living through them is quite another. You, the reader, are the only reason I decided to go back to research, gather current information, interview knowledgeable people on the subject, rewrite, and revise.

Stroke recovery is the most difficult part of my life story. Since I was only 42 years old when the strokes occurred, it happened at the climax of my life. Perhaps that part of my life was either my making or breaking. It wasn't easy. It still isn't easy. But I have learned my particular stroke difficulties and how to overcome most of them. The world keeps spinning, time passes, and life goes on.

For me, many wonderful episodes have been added since stroke. My grandchildren, my graduation from college post-stroke, the books I have authored, the people I have met along the way—these all add up to a full life. Today, I am more readily able to place my personal story in the already written past, and open up new and innovative chapters to help you recover to the best of your ability.

Resources

You and your family are not alone. There are international, national, and community resources available to help you. Here are a few:

American Association of Retired Persons (AARP)
601 E Street NW
Washington, DC 20049
1-800-424-2277
www.aarp.org

American Brain Foundation
201 Chicago Avenue
Minneapolis, MN 55415
1-866-770-7570
www.americanbrainfoundation.org

American Heart Association/American Stroke Association (AHA/ASA)
7272 Greenville Avenue
Dallas, TX 75231-4596
1-888-4-STROKE (1-888-478-7653)
www.strokeassociation.org

American Speech-Language-Hearing Association
10801 Rockville Pike
Rockville, MD 20852
1-800-638-8255
www.asha.org

Bioness Inc.
25134 Rye Canyon Loop, Suite 300
Valencia, CA 91355
(661)-362-4850
www.bioness.com

Bungalow Software, Inc.
(Bungalow offers computer software to assist in recovering speech
and language after stroke.)
1-800-891-9937
http://www.bungalowsoftware.com

Centers for Medicare & Medicaid Services
7500 Security Boulevard
Baltimore, MD 21244-1850
1-800-MEDICARE (1-800-633-4227)
www.medicare.gov

Minnesota Stroke Association
2277 Highway 36 West, Suite 200
Roseville, MN 55113-3830
763-553-0088
www.strokemn.org

Mobility International USA (MIUSA)
132 E. Broadway, Suite 343
Eugene, OR 97401
1-541-343-1284
www.miusa.org

National Aphasia Association
29 John Street, Suite 1103
New York, NY 10038
1-800-922-4622
www.aphasia.org

National Center for Chronic Disease Prevention and Health
Division for Heart Disease and Stroke Prevention
1600 Clifton Road
Atlanta, GA 30329-4027
800-CDC-INFO (800-232-4636)
http://www.cdc.gov/DHDSP

National Institute of Neurological Disorders and Stroke (NINDS)
P.O. Box 5801
Bethesda, MD 20824
1-800-352-9424
www.ninds.nih.gov

National Stroke Association (NSA)
9707 East Easter Lane
Englewood, CO 80112
1-800-STROKES (1-800-787-6563)
www.stroke.org

North Coast Medical, Inc.
8100 Camino Arroyo
Gilroy, CA 95020
(Their catalog *Functional Solutions* can be ordered by calling 1-800-821-9319)
www.ncmedical.com

Saebo, Inc.
Six Lake Pointe Plaza
2709 Water Ridge Pkwy, Suite 100
Charlotte, NC 28217
(888) 284-5433
www.saebo.com

Social Security Administration
Office of Public Inquiries
Windsor Park Building
6401 Security Boulevard
Baltimore, MD 21235
General Information 1-800-772-1213
Enter your zip code to find your local office.
www.socialsecurity.gov
Ticket to Work Program
http://www.ssa.gov/work

Stroke Survivors Association
323 Coventry Road, Unit #72
Ottawa, ON, K1K 3x6 Canada
www.strokesurvivors.ca

The National Library Service (NLS) for the Blind and Physically Handicapped, Library of Congress
1291 Taylor Street, NW
Washington, DC 20542
1-800-424-8567
www.loc.gov/nls
(Also a free program called Braille and Audio Reading Device (BARD) is available through NLS for qualifying participants.)

The Stroke Network
A web-based stroke support and referral organization.
http://www.strokenetwork.org

World Stroke Organization (WSO)
www.world-stroke.org
The WSO is the world's leading organization in the fight against stroke.

Index

About the Author

Cleo Hutton, *Author, Speaker, and Advocate for Stroke Awareness and Recovery Issues*

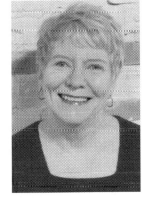

Cleo Hutton authored *After a Stroke: 300 Tips for Making Life Easier*, Demos Medical Publishing, in 2005, and coauthored, with Louis R. Caplan, MD, *Striking Back at Stroke: A Doctor-Patient Journal*, in 2003. She also contributed to the books *Stroke* by Louis R. Caplan, MD, and *Brain Attack, the Journey Back*, edited by Liz Pearl.

Cleo is a 24-year ischemic stroke survivor and has had prior working experience in nursing. Her extensive campaign to spread the word about stroke awareness and recovery has been carried on national radio shows and television broadcasts, including *CNN Health*, and featured in several magazines, including *Prevention, Cerebrum*, and *Stroke Smart*.

Cleo is a compassionate speaker who uses her heart, humor, and experience to deliver a message of hope and healing by breaking paradigms rooted in myths and misconceptions concerning stroke. In 2014, Cleo received the 16th Annual Journey Award from Essentia Health Rehabilitation Services at Essentia Health, Duluth, Minnesota. In 2006, she received Northland News Center's Women in Leadership Award. In 1996, she received the American Heart and Stroke Hero Award.

At the young age of 50, Cleo graduated with honors from the University of Minnesota Duluth with a major in English and a minor in professional writing and communication. She chose these subjects in order to relearn communication and aid comprehension, reading, and writing skills.

The mother of three adult children and a grandmother, Cleo lives in Minnesota with her two Tabby cats, Buddy and Lucy. Cleo is an avid reader who knits and exercises daily. She also volunteers for numerous community services and events.

The name, Cleo Hutton, is a pseudonym for medical and family privacy.